Y0-BVN-998

Future Directions in Infant Development Research

George J. Suci Steven S. Robertson
Editors

Future Directions in Infant Development Research

Springer-Verlag
New York Berlin Heidelberg London Paris
Tokyo Hong Kong Barcelona Budapest

George J. Suci
Steven S. Robertson
Department of Human Development and Family Studies
Cornell University
Ithaca, NY 14853-4401, USA

With 6 Figures.

Library of Congress Cataloging-in-Publication Data
Future directions in infant development research/George J. Suci,
  Steven Robertson, editors.
       p. cm.
     Papers presented at a symposium in honor of Henry Ricciuti,
  sponsored by the College of Human Ecology, Cornell University.
     Includes bibliographical references and index.
     ISBN 0-387-97648-5 (alk. paper)
     1. Infant psychology—Congresses.   2. Infants—Development—
  Congresses.   I. Suci, George J. (George John), 1925–
  II. Robertson, Steven.   III. New York State College of Human
  Ecology.
  BF719.F87   1991
  305.23′2—dc20   91-26407

Printed on acid-free paper.

Production managed by Linda H. Hwang. Manufacturing supervised by
  Jacqui Ashri.
Typeset by Best-set Typesetter Ltd., Hong Kong.
Printed and bound by Braun-Brumfield, Inc., Ann Arbor, MI.
Printed in the United States of America.

9 8 7 6 5 4 3 2 1

ISBN 0-387-97648-5 Springer-Verlag New York Berlin Heidelberg
ISBN 3-540-97648-5 Springer-Verlag Berlin Heidelberg New York

Preface

This book contains the papers presented at a symposium in honor of Henry Ricciuti's promotion to Professor Emeritus in Human Development and Family Studies, a department in the College of Human Ecology at Cornell University. The idea for an event of this kind began in a conversation with Jerome Ziegler, who was then dean of the college. The symposium was conceived as a means for recognizing Henry's many contributions in his roles, both as scholar in the field of human development, and as a member and citizen of this institution. Three of us in the department, Rick Canfield, Steve Robertson, and George Suci, were enthusiastically joined by Henry in a series of planning sessions that resulted in the symposium and the papers in this book. Both Dean Ziegler and Dean Francille Firebaugh generously provided financial support for the symposium.

It was Henry's wish that the focus of the symposium be on the future, that both applied and theoretical perspectives on human development be represented, and that the papers not be bound by any limits on speculation or exploration. The participants chose topics that interesect with the foci of Henry's own work: emotional and cognitive development in infancy and the effects of a variety of factors—nutrition, early interventions, care-giving practices, and social interactions.

The participants were gracious and enthusiastic in accepting our invitation to participate. There was clear consensus about the significance of Henry's contributions in the last 30 years to progress in infancy research, including many "new ventures involving infants and their families" (Joy Osofsky). For example, Henry started an infant day care program in the late 1960s "when many in the field questioned the advisability of taking infants out of the home. . . . The program was important in demonstrating that quality group care for infants can be beneficial, supporting appropriate infant development" (Joy Osofsky). His interest in research with social relevance led him to naturalistic studies well before their popularity in the 1970s. Yet he managed to maintain his characteristic methodological integrity in research conducted outside the tightly controlled conditions of a laboratory, and in fact contributed to the development of new and better observational methods.

The symposium was planned in the spirit of new ventures in both applied and basic research, hence the title of the symposium: Future Directions in Infant Development Research. We hope this will be the first of a series of symposia at Cornell directed at a variety of issues in the development of the human being throughout the life span.

George J. Suci
Steven S. Robertson

Contents

Contributors

Alice Eberhart-Wright
The Menninger Clinic, Box 829, Topeka, KS 66601, USA

Kathleen Gorman
Department of Applied Behavioral Sciences, University of California, Davis, CA 95615, USA

Frances Degen Horowitz
Graduate School and University Center, City University of New York, NY 10036-8099, USA

Jerome Kagan
Department of Psychology, Harvard University, Cambridge, MA 02138, USA

Elizabeth Metallinos-Katsaras
Department of Applied Behavioral Sciences, University of California, Davis, CA 95615, USA

Joy D. Osofsky
Department of Pediatrics; Department of Psychiatry, Louisiana State University Medical Center, New Orleans, LA 70112, USA

Ross D. Parke
Department of Psychology, University of California, Riverside, CA 92521, USA

Ernesto Pollitt
Department of Applied Behavioral Sciences, University of California, Davis, CA 95615, USA

Henry N. Ricciuti
Professor Emeritus, Human Development and Family Studies, College of Human Ecology, Cornell University, Ithaca, NY 14853, USA

Nancy Snidman
Department of Psychology, Harvard University, Cambridge, MA 02138, USA

1
Social Development in Infancy: Looking Backward, Looking Forward

Ross D. Parke

I want to use this opportunity to document and chronicle the significant shifts that have taken place in the field of infant social development from the 1960s to the present—as a way of illustrating both the changes and the progress that we have made and to highlight Henry Ricciuti's role in both anticipating and contributing to this progress. Second, I want to underscore certain trends that I see for the future of research, theory, and methodology in this area.

Let me begin with a brief reminder of the fact that the field of infancy research has matured in the past 20 to 30 years. This is indexed not only by the increase in the rate of publication of articles, chapters, and books that focus on infant social development but also by the creation of specialized groups, organizations, societies, and journals devoted to the topic. In the 1960s the Merrill-Palmer Institute in the United States and the CIBA Foundation in Great Britain sponsored a series of conferences and publications on infancy, including social development (Foss, 1961–1969; Sigel, 1963, 1970). Second, the International Conference on Infant Studies began as a small informal group in 1967 and by the late 1980s was an independent and vigorous organization with regular biennial meetings. Third, new journals such as *Infant Behavior and Development* (1978) and *Infant Mental Health Journal* (1980) made their debut. Finally, the *Handbook of Infant Development* was launched in 1979 and reappeared in a second edition in 1987 (Osofsky, 1979, 1987). All of these indicators bear witness to the emergence of the field of infancy research in this period.

1

As we highlight the recent trends in our field, it is important to remember that certain questions and issues are ever present. What has changed is our emphasis and our way of addressing these issues. In this essay, I will do two things. First, I will comment on some topics that I see as emerging as areas of more intense activity. Second, I will try to show how our views of some long-standing concerns and issues have changed.

To anticipate, I will argue (a) that we are recognizing the inter-dependence across domains, (b) that development needs to be viewed as a series of interacting trajectories, and (c) that we need to pay closer attention to long-standing issues of sampling.

The Emergence of New Themes

Emotional Development

Perhaps the most dramatic shift in content-based interest in the last 25 years has been the renewal of interest in the development of emotions in infancy. Topics such as social smiling, stranger anxiety, and fear of heights were of interest in the 1960s (Gibson & Walk, 1960; Spitz, 1950), but "the motivation for conducting such studies was to use emotions to index something else—usually perceptual or cognitive process" (Campos, Barrett, Lamb, Goldsmith, & Sternberg, 1983, p. 786). The development of emotions and the role of emotions in social interaction were of little interest. A dramatic change has occurred. Throughout psychology the role of affect became an issue of increasing concern in the 1980s (e.g., Zajonc, Murphy, & Inglehart, 1989). The developmental origins of both the production and recognition of emotions as well as the role of emotional expressions in the regulation of social interaction continue to be central concerns of developmental psychologists, especially infancy researchers.

Under the guidance of the research and writings of Ekman (Ekman & Friesen, 1978) and of Izard (1982), the older assumption that facial response patterns are not specific to discrete emotional states is being discounted. Evidence suggests that facial expressions may be, at least in part, governed by genetically encoded pro-grams—an implication of the finding of universality of facial expression recognition (Ekman & Friesen, 1978).

The shift toward recognition of the role of emotional expressions in the regulation of social behavior is one of the most important shifts in recent years (e.g., Camaras, 1977). The extensive studies of face-to-face interaction of parents and infants (e.g., Brazelton, Koslowski, & Main, 1974; Stern, 1977, 1985) illustrate how parents and possibly infants modify their patterns of stimulation in response to each other's emotional signals.

One of the ways in which the social regulatory effects of emotions has been demonstrated is through the notion of "social referencing" (Campos & Stenberg, 1981). Social referencing concerns the tendency of a person to seek out emotional information from a significant other in the environment and to use that information to make sense of an event that is otherwise ambiguous or beyond the person's own intrinsic appraisal capabilities (Campos & Stenbery, 1981). Investigators have shown that infants' reactions to novel toys (Klinnert, 1981); the visual cliff (Sorce, Emde, Klinnert, & Campos, 1981); and adult strangers (Feinman & Lewis, 1981) can be modified by the nature of the mother's facial expressions, with positive expressions (such as happiness) eliciting approach behavior and negative emotional displays (such as fear) leading to avoidance. Moreover, social referencing is sensitive to the prior relationship that the infant has established with the referencing agent—a further index of the close ties between emotions and social relationships (Dickstein & Parke, 1988, 1990).

It is evident that there has been a clear resurgence of interest in various aspects of emotional development in infancy, including the role of emotions in the regulation of social behavior.

Biological Basis of Infant Social Behavior

A further development of considerable importance is the increasing interest in the biological underpinnings of social behavior in infancy as well as in adolescence. This development assumes a variety of forms. One form is interest in the patterning of psychophysiological responses associated with either different emotions or different social situations, such as separation from the mother or entry of a stranger (Field, 1987). These studies provide further evidence in support of the specificity of emotion hypothesis as well as another index of emotional responsivity in different situations.

A second manifestation of the recent upsurge of interest in biology is the renewed interest in behavioral genetics. This work has generally taken the form of determining the possible genetic origins of certain traits, such as extraversion and introversion, as well as the age of onset of emotional markers, such as smiling and fear of strangers. Recently, Plomin and DeFries (1985) found that identical twins exhibit greater concordance than fraternal twins in the time of onset and in the amount of social smiling. Similarly, identical twins are more similar in social responsiveness than fraternal twins (Plomin, 1986).

Social Relationships

A third theme is the continuing interest in social interactive processes and the ways in which these face-to-face processes emerge into the *formation of social relationships* (Hartup & Rubin, 1986; Hinde, 1979). Moreover, there is an increasing appreciation of the range of characters who play a prominent role. Our definition of family has expanded to include a focus not only on the mother-infant dyad but on the role of fathers, siblings, and grandparents in infant social development as well (Dunn & Kendrick, 1982; Parke & Tinsley, 1987; Tinsley & Parke, 1987).

Finally, there is a growing appreciation of the embeddedness of families in a variety of social systems outside the family, including peer, school, and kin-based networks (Bronfenbrenner, 1986; Cochran & Brassard, 1979; Parke & Ladd, 1992).

Shifts in Content-Free Dimensions of Infant Social Development

Shifts in Theoretical Orientation: Explanatory Models

The study of infant social development can be characterized by the types of models of development endorsed by theorists. According to Overton and Reese (1973), these rival models were termed mechanistic and organismic world views or models and more recently as scientific research programs. The importance of these views flows from the assumption that the choice of explanatory models determines a variety of theoretical decisions and the nature of testable hypotheses.

The 1960s were dominated by the mechanistic model, although the organismic viewpoint also had advocates. Proponents of behavioristic or neobehavioristic theorists (Gewirtz, 1965; Lipsitt, 1963; Rheingold, 1956) were active scientific leaders and producers. Similarly, social learning theories (Bandura & Walters, 1963) predominated in the period, but with some exceptions. Piaget's theory was beginning to be influential (Flavell, 1963) in American psychology, and Kessen (1967), in particular, offered an organismic analysis of infant development.

The situation in the 1980s and 1990s has changed, with various versions of an organismic viewpoint clearly predominating. In the domain of social development, Bowlby's ethologically oriented attachment theory is a major force (Ainsworth, 1973; Sroufe & Fleeson, 1986). A second major theoretical development of current importance is the ecological perspective of Bronfenbrenner (1979, 1986). This viewpoint has been applied to the infancy domain by Belsky (1984) and is consistent with another general trend toward a systems theory viewpoint (Belsky, Rovine, & Fish, 1989; Ramey, MacPhee, & Yeates, 1982; Sameroff, 1983). All of these views are clearly organismic in orientation. The 1990s clearly belong to the organismically oriented theories.

Types of Principal Explanatory Processes

Every era is characterized by different sets of explanatory principles or processes that serve as the centerpiece for explaining the emergence and maintenance of behavior under question. These include biological, cognitive, affective, perceptual, learning, and social interactional processes. Although in every era some attention is obviously paid to all of these processes, some generally preferred processes gain prominence in different periods of investigation. Major shifts have occurred in the processes involved in explaining infant social behavior over the past quarter century.

First, the 1960s era was characterized by a major focus on perceptual, sensory, and learning processes (Lipsitt, 1963). In the realm of social development, the same learning principles predominated in the early 1960s. One group of researchers (e.g., Gewirtz, 1965; Rheingold, 1956) believed that contingent reinforcement from social agents shapes the form and frequency of social responses such as smiling and vocalizing. Closely related were social interactionists, who believed that similar processes operated under naturalistic conditions (e.g., Schaffer & Emerson, 1964).

The 1980s are more eclectic in terms of the processes that are drawn upon to explain social developmental changes in infancy. Current explanations draw upon a wide range of explanatory processes. First, biological processes are given more recognition, including concepts of preparedness to respond to social events and concepts of individual differences in temperament, as well as notions of genetic determination of the forms of social and affective behavior (Bates, 1987; Plomin, 1986; Schaffer, 1984). Second, affective processes are viewed as important modifiers of infant social (and cognitive) development (Campos et al., 1983). Third, both perceptual and cognitive processes are invoked to explain the occurrence of social behaviors (Campos et al., 1983). Fourth, social interactional processes have been given a central explanatory role in the emergence and maintenance of social behavior (Parke & Tinsley, 1987; Schaffer, 1984). The diversity of explanatory processes is one of the hallmarks of the 1980s era.

Aims of Theory

Theories across various disciplines vary in terms of their goals. Within developmental psychology, ethological (Blurton-Jones, 1972) and ecological approaches (Barker, 1968) are largely descriptive. Others are aimed at increasing the level of predictability of behavior and/or modifying the extent to which behavior can be brought under control. Skinnerian approaches as well as behavior modification theories (Bijou & Baer, 1961) have prediction and control as their primary goals. Finally, explanation is the goal of the grand theories of Freud and Piaget as well as recent theories of infant social development such as Bowlby's attachment theory (Bowlby, 1969–1980).

Within the domain of infant social development, the relative emphasis on these three theoretical goals has shifted. In the 1960s, a great deal of research activity was devoted to the study of the factors that could exercise control over infants' social behavior, such as smiling and vocalizing (e.g., Gewirtz, 1965). The goals of description and explanation received less attention.

In the intervening period, concern with both description and explanation has increased. A primary goal of Bowlby's attachment theory was to provide a descriptive account of the ways in which children manage the naturally occurring events of separation and loss. Similarly, the goal of recent ethologically influenced studies of the emergence of emotional expressiveness in infancy has been largely descriptive (e.g., Izard & Malatesta, 1987). The ecological orientation of Bronfenbrenner (1979) has led to an increased concern with a description of social contexts and settings that infants may encounter during development. A large portion of the activity of the 1970s and 1980s in the area of parent-infant interaction has been descriptive. Description of changes in parent-infant interaction as a function of developmental level of the infant, task, and context has been the primary goal of this research activity (see Maccoby & Martin, 1983; Osofsky, 1987).

However, implicit in this work has been the assumption that description is a first step in a multistage process. Explanation follows as a next step in theory development. Explanatory theories of infant social development have emerged and range from psychoanalytically oriented positions (Mahler & Pine, 1975), to psychoanalytic-ethological (Bowlby, 1969), to family systems theory (Lewis, 1982) and transactional positions (Sameroff & Chandler, 1975).

This shift back to an emphasis on descriptive as well as analytic studies was anticipated by Henry Ricciuti in the late 1960s.

Early studies of social and emotional behavior in infancy tended to be primarily descriptive in nature. . . . The major historical change . . . has been the transition from the descriptive focus to the contemporary emphasis on analytic studies. . . . While it has become somewhat fashionable in recent years to speak rather disparagingly of studies which are primarily descriptive in nature, I would like to emphasize the very real impact of these early studies which provided so many insightful observations and questions concerning social and emotional behavior. (Ricciuti, 1968, p. 83)

Scope of Our Theories

A major difference in the field now, and hopefully in the future, is that our era of compartmentalization is slowly passing. We have passed through two phases.

A gradual shift has occurred in the scope of our theories. Theorists in the grand tradition of Freud, Piaget, and more recently the social learning theorists (Bandura & Walters, 1963) assumed that very large domains of social or cognitive development could be accounted for in terms of a limited number of general principles. As Kessen (1982) has observed, "At an accelerated rate, child psychologists as a Society of colleagues have moved away from the general process, general-principle specification of their intellectual task. More and more we have turned from the search for singular general laws of development" (p. 36). In the past 25 to 30 years, the degree of specialization has increased sharply; in place of grand theories, a variety of minitheories aimed at limited and specific aspects of development have emerged. In the domain of infant social development, theories and research have been devoted to the emergence of infant-parent attachments (Ainsworth, 1973); father-infant relationships (Lamb, 1981; Parke, 1981); and the emergence of and measurement of affect in infants (Izard & Malatesta, 1987). Each of these theoretical developments is highly restricted in its scope and explanatory area. Similar trends are evident in cognitive development (Flavell, 1985).

However, there are strands of evidence that we are recognizing that this isolation of minitheories may not be appropriate. There is a recognition that the domains of childhood—social, emotional, physical, health, and cognitive aspects—are interdependent, and it is recognized that they overlap and mutually influence each other.

Consider the following prophetic quote from Ricciuti:

We cannot adequately study social and emotional behavior in infancy independently of other basic psychological processes involved in the infant's behavior and development. Perceptual-cognitive and learning processes clearly play a major role in determining what social and emotional responses will be elicited by particular stimulus conditions, as well as how such responses will be expressed in behavior. . . . Conversely, social and emotional factors play a significant role in the development of perceptual-cognitive behavior and of various motivational systems. One of the significant features of the contemporary research scene is that many investigators are increasingly inclined to examine the role of the *various* psychological processes which may be involved in particular transactions of importance between the infant and his environment. (1968, p. 97)

To illustrate that this call for more porous boundaries between domains has, in fact, been partially realized, consider the following examples.

First, there is a rise in interest in the interplay between social and cognitive development, especially in how social input (e.g., scaffolding) on the part of the mother can increase the level of cognitive performance of children. The reemergence of interest in Vygotskian theory is one form of this interest (Rogoff, 1990).

Second, and closely related, is the increase in interest in the role of cognitive factors in the explanation of social processes. For example, the recent work on "working models" within the attachment paradigm is a search for a explanation of how the expectations and social rules acquired in the context of the parent-child relationship become guides or maps that the child imposes on other social relationships (Bretherton & Waters, 1985).

Third, the ways in which temperament—an index of biological predispositions—interacts with social contextual variables in affecting child outcome (e.g., Crockenberg, 1981) is a further example of the interplay across domains.

Fourth, recent work on language, communication, and perceptual development is often studied in the context of social development (Bruner, 1983; Nelson, 1987).

Finally, Henry Ricciuti's own work on the interplay between malnutrition and cognitive development is a further example of the fact that the barriers between domains of developmental inquiry are eroding (Ricciuti, 1970, 1980).

Toward Interdisciplinary Research and Dialogue

Not only are barriers falling across content domains within our own discipline, but a rise in interdisciplinary cooperation is evident as well. In comparison to the 1960s, there is a variety of indications of a marked increase in interdisciplinary cooperation. This is evident in links with pediatrics in both training (Parmalee, 1982; Tinsley & Parke, 1984) and research (Goldberg & DeVitto, 1983; Ricciuti & Breitmayer, 1988). Second, due to the rise of interest in developmental psychopathology, collaboration between child psychiatry and developmental researchers has increased (Sameroff & Emde, 1989). Third, there are increased links with sociology and psychology as indexed by collaborative work on day care, divorce, and timing of parenthood (e.g., Furstenberg, Brooks-Gunn, & Morgan, 1987; Hoffreth & Phillips, 1987). Fourth, geneticists, neurologists, and psychophysiologists are all prominent collaborators with infant researchers in the 1980s (Gunnar, 1987; Plomin, 1986). Finally, developmentalists and historians are increasingly aware of each other (Elder, Modell, & Parke, 1992). The 1980s and 90s represent a rich context for interdisciplinary research in infant social development.

Universal Versus Culturally and Historically Based Explanations

In the 1960s, it was widely assumed that our theories were universally applicable, and relatively little attention was paid to contributions of culture to our explanations. In the 1970s and 1980s, more attention was paid to cross-cultural work in the domain of infant social development (Field, Sostek, Vietze, &

Leiderman, 1981; Kagan & Klein, 1973). These studies have served as important reminders that the generalizations concerning infant social development derived from studies of American samples may, in fact, not be valid in some other cultural contexts.

This is not news to Ricciuti, who has long appreciated the need for cultural sensitivity in terms of our conclusions but also recognizes that cultural contexts present the opportunity for natural experiments. For example, the studies of malnutrition that he has carried out in Peru and India are witness to the value of cross-cultural research for our understanding of basic processes (Ricciuti, 1973, 1983).

Closely related to the increased sensitivity to cross-cultural variations is an increase in recognition of the importance of *historical* context for interpreting our findings about infant social development (Elder, 1984). The recent rise of interest in infant day care is clearly viewed through a historically sensitive lens (Clarke-Stewart, 1989; Ricciuti & Thomas, 1989).

Applied Versus Nonapplied Orientation

In spite of a long-standing commitment to the application of knowledge about development to solving applied problems, in the 1960s researchers showed less interest in these issues. However, in the 1980s several trends converged to redirect our attention to applied concerns. First, the nature of our research problems has shifted toward an increased emphasis on mental health and social relevance (Sroufe & Rutter, 1984). Second, our populations have changed to a focus on at-risk infants such as premature babies and handicapped babies, as well as at-risk parent groups such as poor and young mothers (Field, 1987). Third, research settings shifted to include hospitals, institutions, and day-care centers. Fourth, such large-scale intervention projects such as Head Start have shifted their focus to the earliest years of development. Finally, there is a rise of interest in the application of research for guiding our formation of social policy (Stevenson & Siegal, 1984).

These shifts come as no surprise to Ricciuti, who has maintained a long-standing commitment to both applied and basic research and has always appreciated the mutual benefits that each approach can have for the other strategy. Witness his research on malnutrition (Ricciuti, 1970); day care (Willis & Ricciuti, 1975); and social policy (Caldwell & Ricciuti, 1973) over the past 2 decades.

The Multiple Phases of Development: Beyond Critical Periods

Each era can be characterized in terms of the period of development that is emphasized. From the 1960s to the present, the infancy period has been rediscovered as an important phase of development. Other periods, especially middle childhood and adolescence, are beginning to challenge the emphasis on infancy, but the treatment of infancy as an isolated period of development is beinning to shift.

Researchers in the late 1980s were coming to take seriously the view of infancy within a life-span perspective (Baltes, 1987). In part, this view emerges from a recognition that the social context provided by caregivers varies as a function of the location of the adults along their own life course trajectory (Parke, 1988). In contrast, the earlier view was that variations in parenting behavior are relatively independent of adult development. Evidence of this shift comes from a variety of sources, including studies of the impact of the timing of parenthood and the effects of maternal (and paternal) employment, job satisfaction, and involvement on infant development (see Parke & Tinsley, 1984, 1987, for reviews).

In summary, by a reconceptualization of the family context in a life-span perspective, the infancy period itself is relocated in a longer time frame that goes well beyond the narrow age boundaries of the first few years of development.

Consistent with this shift toward a life-span view is the reevaluation of role of critical periods in development. In the 1960s, considerable evidence supported the critical period hypothesis as it related to infant social development. Several lines of research converged in support of this viewpoint from both animal (e.g., Harlow & Harlow, 1962; Sackett, 1968) and human (Yarrow, 1961, 1964) studies.

However, since the 1960s important challenges have been mounted that bring into serious question the critical period hypothesis in regard to the development of infant social behavior. First, later research seriously challenged one of the central postulates of a critical period view of development, namely, that certain periods of development are of particular importance and that the individual who does not receive an appropriate experience during this phase will suffer permanent deficits. Research has strongly challenged this view by showing that monkeys reared in total social isolation for the first 6 months of life can be rehabilitated (Novak & Harlow,

1975). Similarly, evidence at the human level has continued to accumulate and challenge the assumption of nonreversibility (Clarke & Clarke, 1976; Kagan & Klein, 1973).

A similar conclusion is evident from more recent studies of infant-parent attachment. A variety of studies have shown that early attachment relationships show a high level of stability across the first few years of life (Sroufe & Fleeson, 1986). However, other evidence suggests that the classification of attachment in infancy shifts across time as a result of changes in family circumstances (Lamb, Thompson, Gardner, Charnov, & Estes, 1984). These findings illustrate the modifiability of attachment relationships.

The Individual Versus Other Units of Analysis

Every era can be characterized by the units of analysis that are preferred for empirical and theoretical work. Individuals, dyads, triads, and polyadic units such as families are possible units that can be utilized. The 1960s and 1980s show marked contrasts in the choice of the unit of analysis.

Accounts of psychological development have for the most part been individually based. Their concern has been with the child as such; it is the child who is regarded as the basic unit of study, everything outside his skin being considered extraneous, even antithetical—forces that may have an impact on the child but that are not an inherent part of his developmental progress. (Schaffer, 1984, p. 11)

This description captures well the 1960s and 1970s, when the unit of analysis was generally the individual. Typically, the infant was examined in order to assess his or her response to input from social agents in the environment. The unit was not simply the individual but often only the infant. Adults, of course, should be expected to behave differently toward infants as a function of their own developmental progress. However, researchers typically had little interest in how the adult social agents who populate an infant's world change developmentally, or in how their developmental changes shape the form and frequency of the social input they provide to infants. They were interested in the effects of different kinds of child-rearing practices (Sears, Maccoby, & Levin, 1957) but had little interest in the reasons for individual differences across adults in their choices of practices. Shifts in family circumstances, life events, occupational changes, or even simply age differences across adults were rarely examined. The 1960s was an individual-istic and infant-oriented period. Moreover, units of analysis beyond the individual were seldom investigated and were rarely the object even of theoretical inquiry.

In the 1980s, a variety of changes occurred. First, researchers now have an increased appreciation of adult development and of how shifts in adult development shape the course of the adult role as socializer of the infant's development (Elder, 1984; Parke, 1988). This expansion of the cast of individuals from the infant to the adult was encouraged, in part by the life-span developmental theorists (Baltes, 1987). However, this expansion merely laid the groundwork for the movement from an individual to a dyadic level of analysis, in that the limiting of our analysis of infant social development to individual development even when both child and adult developmental trajectories are considered is viewed as inadequate.

In the 1980s, researchers began to conceptualize the unit of analysis as dyads within the family system such as the parent-child dyad, the husband-wife dyad, and the sib-sib dyad (Belsky, 1984; Cowan et al., 1985, Parke, 1988; Parke & Tinsley, 1987). Moreover, units beyond the dyad have been recognized as important as well. Infant research models that limit examination of the effects of interaction patterns to only the father-infant and mother-infant dyads and the direct effects of one individual on another are now assumed to be inadequate for understanding the impact of social interaction patterns in families (Belsky, 1984; Kreppner, 1988; Parke, Power, & Gottman, 1979; Pedersen, 1980). Several re-searchers have recently begun to investigate triads (Hinde & Stevenson-Hinder, 1988; Kreppner, 1988) as well as the family as units of analysis (Reiss, 1981). It is clear that units of analysis that extend beyond the individual were increasingly recognized in the late 1980s (Parke, 1988; Sigel & Parke, 1987).

Moreover, these various units of analysis may each follow sep-arate and possibly disparate developmental pathways. The task of tracing the developmental trajectory of the individual child or adult is only one challenge of the 1980s and 90s; an equally important agenda is to evaluate the developmental trajectory followed by different dyads (mother-infant, sib-sib, mother-father); triads (father-sib-sib, mother-father-child); or family units (mother-father-children). Moreover, the interplay among these separate develop-mental trajectories can produce a diverse set of effects on the functioning of the units themselves. Both the timing and nature of developmentally linked change will be determined by the points at which particular individuals, dyads, triads, and families fall along their respective developmental trajectories. Individual families can vary widely in terms of the particular configuration of the life course pathways. The timing of the onset of parenthood is associated with a wide array of different effects for individual infants, as well as parent-child and marital dyads (Brooks-Gunn & Furstenberg, 1986; Parke, 1988), as well as family units (Walter, 1986). Briefly, both the father-infant dyad may be stronger and the marital dyad more stable in late versus early timed parenthood families, which, in turn, alters the nature of the infant's early social context. (See Parke, 1988, for a detailed analysis of this issue.) The central premise is that the particular configuration of these multiple sets of developmental trajectories needs to be considered in order to fully understand the nature of infant social development. The 1980s witnessed our shift toward more complex units of analysis in contrast to our earlier preoccupation with the individual. The challenge of the 1990s is to conceptualize and investigate the developmental implications of this expansion of our units of analysis. To do this we need to develop theories that account for the multiple developmental trajectories followed by various units of analysis.

Shifts in Our Methodological Orientation

In addition to shifts in our theoretical assumptions, the past three decades have witnessed a variety of shifts in our methodological approaches to infant social development. Several changes can be briefly highlighted. First, there is an increased commitment to both longitudinal research designs and cross-sectional approaches. Second, in contrast to the dominance of experimental approaches in the 1960s, the 1980s were characterized by an openness to multiple strategies, including lab-based experimental studies and a variety of nonexperimental approaches (Parke, 1989). Third, the research settings have changed from a near exclusive focus on the lab context in the 1960s to an increased utilization of natural contexts for the conduct of research (Bronfenbrenner, 1979).

Selection of Samples

An important change has taken place in our choice of samples. In the 1960s, we were satisfied with our highly selected nonrepresentative samples, in part due to our focus on the search for experimentally derived process-oriented laws of early social development. A variety of conditions have conspired to increase our awareness of the limitations of samples, including our awareness of cultural and historical diversity, as well as the increasing interest in testing multivariate models of development.

These shifts in our awareness regarding sampling issues have led to an increase in interest in large representative national samples. Although this has typically been the domain of sociologists and survey researchers, developmentalists in the early 1990s are showing an increased awareness of the potential value of supplementing their usual small-sample strategies with these large-sample approaches. The most prominent example is the rise in the use of the National Longitudinal Study of Youth (NLSY) for the examination of a variety of developmental issues, including divorce, achievement, and day care (Brooks-Gunn, Phelps, & Elder, in press). These surveys have several advantages, including the large number of subjects, more representative samples, the multifaceted range of variables, and the longitudinal nature of the design. In turn, these characteristics permit us to test more complex models of development that require large numbers of subjects. In addition, these studies allow examination of connections across content-based domains, as well as encouraging and permiting interdisciplinary cooperation. Finally, they permit us to test the cultural generality of our models.

It should be underscored that these approaches are not free of methodological limitations. Often the measures are limited to only a few items that must be relied upon to operationalize the construct of interest. Moreover, the impact of repeated testing may present problems. In addition, the reliance on easily administered tests, which are often based on self-reports, may limit the value of these approaches. However, recent waves of the NLSY have included a variety of cognitive and social measures that are based on observed performance rather than self-reports. In any case, the increased utilization of these large-scale data bases was a new and emerging trend in the 1980s and will likely continue throughout the present decade.

Newer, more innovative approaches that combine levels of sampling are becoming increasingly common as well. As a supplement to a large-scale survey approach, researchers are selecting a subsample of subjects for more intensive examination of particular process of interest. Two examples will illustrate. Recently, Bietel and Parke (1990) conducted a survey of 300 families to assess maternal attitudes toward father involvement in infant care. To supplement this approach, in which a self-report questionnaire was employed, a subsample of 40 families were observed in their homes as a way to validate the self-report data. Similarly, Reiss, Hetherington, and Plomin (1990) have generated a nationally representative sample of stepfamilies, and in a second stage of their work, they have observed these families in interaction tasks in the home. These combined approaches increase both the generalizability of our findings and at the same time allow us to illuminate basic social processes.

Conclusion

This historical voyage over the past 3 decades of the field of infant social development and of Henry Ricciuti's role in this changing field has revealed a variety of shifts in the conceptual under-pinnings that serve to guide research and theory in this domain. As I have noted throughout this essay, many of these shifts were anticipated by Henry Ricciuti in his own work and writings. Several features of these shifts are noteworthy.

The field is more eclectic and open in the early 1990s than in the 1960s in terms of the variety of theories, contexts, and methods that characterize the field. A new sensitivity to the issues of cultural and historical variations is evident in both our theories and in our choice of samples.

Infant social development is viewed at present in a life-span developmental perspective, which has led us to an expanded view of not only the appropriate time frame for developmental analysis but also to a richer cast of family players and units of study.

Another feature of this shift has been the movement away from the grand theories of the 1960s (Freud, Hull-Spence, Piaget) and to the emergence of a series of domain specific minitheories that aim to explain smaller pieces of the developmental puzzle. A new stage was noted, namely the emergence of cross-domain and cross-disciplinary integrations. These signs of integration and dialogue may represent the early steps toward a new phase in the form of a systems perspective that holds promise of uniting biological, social, cognitive, and emotional minitheories into a more unified and coherent framework. Several recent efforts in the 1980s suggest that this move to a middle-level theoretical ground is a promising development for the field (Fogel & Thelen, 1987; Sameroff, 1983). A recent volume of the *Minnesota Symposium on Child Psychology* (Gunnar, 1989) was devoted to the utility of a systems perspective in accounting for various aspects of development. It remains to be seen whether this represents a useful direction for our theoretical work or whether with this move to a further level of abstraction and generality, we will lose the richness and specificity that led us to retreat to minitheories and domain-specific theories in the first place. At this stage, it seems worth the effort, particularly since there are no signs of the imminent emergence of a new Freud or Piaget!

In conclusion, I end on a note of optimism, since it is evident that we are beginning to appreciate once again the interplay across systems and the complexity of the infant's social environment. Moreover, with our new openness in terms of our samples and methods, not only will our data be richer, but our understanding of process and the generalizability of our findings will be clearer as well.

References

Ainsworth, M.D.S. (1973). The development of infant-mother attachment. In B. Caldwell & H. Ricciuti (Eds.), *Review of child development research* (Vol. 3). Chicago: University of Chicago Press.

Baltes, P.B. (1987). Theoretical propositions of life span developmental psychology: On the dynamics of growth and decline. *Developmental Psychology, 23*, 611–626.

Bandura, A., & Walters, R.H. (1963). *Social learning and personality development.* New York: Holt, Rinehart & Winston.

Barker, R.G. (1968). *Ecological psychology: Concepts and methods for studying the environment of human behavior.* Stanford, CA: Stanford University Press.

Bates, J.E. (1987). Temperament in infancy. In J.D. Osofsky (Ed.), *Handbook of infant development* (2nd ed., pp. 1101–1149). New York: Wiley.

Belsky, J. (1984). The determinants of parenting: A process model. *Child Development, 55*, 83–96.

Belsky, J., Rovine, M., & Fish, M. (1989). The developing family system. In M. Gunnar (Ed.), *Minnesota symposium in child psychology* (Vol. 22). Hillsdale, NJ: Erlbaum.

Bietel, A., & Parke, R.D. (1990). The role of maternal attitudes in father involvement with infants. Unpublished manuscript, University of Illinois.

Bijou, S.W., & Baer, D.M. (1961). *Child development: A systematic and empirical theory* (Vol. 1). New York: Appleton-Century-Crofts.

Blurton Jones, N. (Ed.) (1972). *Ethological studies of child behavior.* Cambridge, England: Cambridge University Press.

Bowlby, J. (1969–1980). *Attachment and loss* (Vols. 1–3) London: Hogarth Press.

Brazelton, T.B., Koslowski, B., & Main, M. (1974). The origins of reciprocity: Early mother-infant interaction. In M. Lewis & L.A. Rosenblum (Eds.), *The effect of the infant on its caregiver.* New York: Wiley.

Bretherton, I., & Waters, E. (Eds.). (1985). Growing points in attachment. *Monographs of the Society for Research in Child Development, 50,* Nos. 1–2, Serial No. 209.

Bronfenbrenner, U. (1979). *The ecology of human development.* Cambridge, MA: Harvard University Press.

Bronfenbrenner, U. (1986). Ecology of the family as a context for human development: Research perspectives. *Developmental Psychology, 22,* 723–742.

Brooks-Gunn, J., & Furstenberg, F.F. (1986). The children of adolescent mothers: Physical, academic and psychological outcomes. *Developmental Review, 6,* 224–251.

Brooks-Gunn, J., Phelps, E., & Elder, G.H. (in press). Studying lives through time: Secondary data analysis in developmental psychology. *Developmental Psychology, 27.*

Bruner, J. (1983). *Children's talk.* New York: Norton.

Caldwell, B.M., & Ricciuti, H.N. (Eds.). (1973). *Review of child development research, Vol. 3: Child development and social policy.* Chicago: University of Chicago Press.

Camaras, L.A. (1977). Facial expression used by children in a conflict situation. *Child Development, 48,* 1431–1435.

Campos, J.J., Barrett, K.C., Lamb, M.E., Goldsmith, H.H., & Sternberg, C. (1983). Socioemotional development. In M.M. Haith & J.J. Campos (Eds.), *Handbook of child psychology, Vol. 2: Infancy and developmental psychobiology* (pp. 783–916). New York: Wiley.

Campos, J.J., & Stenberg, C.R. (1981). Perception, appraisal and emotion: The onset of social referencing. In M.E. Lamb & L.R. Sherrod (Eds.), *Infant social cognition: Empirical and theoretical considerations.* Hillsdale, NJ: Erlbaum.

Clarke, A.M., & Clarke, A.D.B. (1976). *Early experience: Myth and evidence.* London: Open Books.

Clarke-Stewart, A.K. (1989). Infant day care: Maligned or malignant? *American Psychologist, 44,* 266–273.

Cochran, M.M., & Brassard, J.A. (1979). Child development and personal social networks. *Child Development, 50,* 601–616.

Cowan, C.P., Cowan, P.A., Heming, G., Garrett, E.V., Coysh, W.S., Curtis-Boles, H., & Boles, A.J. (1985). Transitions to parenthood: His, hers and theirs. *Journal of Family Issues, 6,* 451–481.

Crockenberg, S.B. (1981). Infant irritability, mother responsiveness, and social support influences on the security of infant-mother attachment. *Child Development, 52,* 857–865.

Dickstein, S., & Parke, R.D. (1988). Social referencing: A glance at fathers and marriage. *Child Development, 59,* 506–511.

Dickstein, S., & Parke, R.D. (1990, April). Infant social referencing: Impact of marital satisfaction and family of origin relationships. Paper presented at the International Conference on Infant Studies, Montreal, Canada.

Dunn, J., & Kendrick, C. (1982). *Siblings: Love, envy and understanding.* Cambridge, MA: Harvard University Press.

Ekman, P., & Friesen, W. (1978). *Facial action coding system.* Palo Alto, CA: Consulting Psychological Press.

Elder, G.H. (1984). Families, kin and the life course: A sociological perspective. In R.D. Parke, R.N. Emde, H.P. McAdoo, & G.P. Sackett (Eds.), *Review of child development research: The family* (Vol. 7, pp. 80–136). Chicago: University of Chicago Press.

Elder, G.H., Modell, J., & Parke, R.D. (Eds.). (1992). *Children in time and place.* New York: Cambridge University Press.

Feinman, S., & Lewis, M. (1981, April). Social referencing and second-order effects in 10-month-old infants. Paper presented at the meeting of the Society of Research in Child Development, Boston, Massachusetts.

Field, T.M. (1987). Affective and interactive processes in disturbed infants. In J.D. Osofsky (Ed.), *Handbook of infant development* (2nd ed., pp. 972–1005). New York: Wiley.

Field, T.M., Sostek, A.M., Vietze, P., & Liederman, P.H. (Eds.). (1981). *Culture and social interactions.* Hillsdale, NJ: Erlbaum.

Flavell, J. (1963). *The developmental psychology of Jean Piaget.* New York: Van Nostrand Reinhold.

Flavell, J. (1985). *Cognitive development* (2nd ed.). Englewood Cliffs, NJ: Prentice-Hall.

Fogel, A., & Thelen, E. (1987). Development of early expressive and communicative action: Reinterpreting the evidence from a dynamic systems perspective. *Developmental Psychology, 23,* 747–761.

Foss, B.M. (Ed.) (1961–1969). *Determinants of infant behavior* (Vols. 1–4). London: Methuen.

Furstenberg, F.F., Brooks-Gunn, J., & Morgan, P. (1987). *Adolescent mothers in later life.* New York: Cambridge University Press.

Gewirtz, J.L. (1965). The course of infant smiling in four child-rearing environmments in Israel. In B.M. Foss (Ed.), *Determinants of infant behavior,* Vol. 3 (pp. 205–248). London: Methuen.

Gibson, E.J., & Walk, R.R. (1960). The "visual cliff." *Scientific American, 202*, 2–9.

Goldberg, S., & DeVitto, B.A. (1983). *Born too soon.* San Francisco, CA: Freeman.

Gunnar, M.R. (1987). Psychological studies of stress and coping: An introduction. *Child Development, 58*, 1403–1407.

Gunnar, M.R. (Ed.). (1989). *Minnesota symposium on child psychology,* Vol. 22. Hillsdale, NJ: Erlbaum.

Harlow, H.F., & Harlow, M.K. (1962). Social deprivation in monkeys. *Scientific American, 207*, 137–146.

Hartup, W.W., & Rubin, Z. (Eds.). (1986). *Relationships and development.* Hillsdale, NJ: Erlbaum.

Hinde, R.A. (1979). *Towards understanding relationships.* London: Academic Press.

Hinde, R.A., & Stevenson-Hinde, J. (1988). *Relationships within families: Mutual influences.* Oxford: Oxford University Press.

Hoffreth, S.L., & Phillips, D.A. (1987). Child care in the United States, 1970 to 1995. *Journal of Marriage and the Family, 49*, 559–572.

Izard, C.E. (1982). *Measuring emotions in infants and children.* New York: Cambridge University Press.

Izard, C.E., & Malatesta, C.Z. (1987). Perspectives on emotional development, I: Differential emotions theory of early emotional development. In J.D. Osofsky (Ed.), *Handbook of infant development* (2nd ed., pp. 494–554). New York: Wiley.

Kagan, J., & Klein, R. (1973). Cross-cultural perspectives on early development. *American Psychologist, 28*, 947–961.

Kessen, W. (1982). The child and other cultural inventions. In F.S. Kessel & A.W. Siegel (Eds.), *The child and other cultural inventions* (pp. 26–39). New York: Praeger.

Kessen, W. (1967). Sucking and looking: Two organized patterns of behavior in the human newborn. In H.W. Stevenson, E.H. Hess, & H.C. Rheingold (Eds.), *Early behavior: Comparative & developmental approaches* (pp. 147–179). New York: Wiley.

Klinnert, M.D. (1981, April). Infants' use of mothers' facial expressions for regulating their own behavior. Presented at the meeting of the Society for Research in Child Development, Boston, Massachusetts.

Kreppner, K. (1988). Changes in dyadic relationships within a family after the arrival of a second child. In R. Hinde & J. Stevenson-Hinde (Eds.), *Relationships within families.* London: Cambridge University Press.

Lamb, M.E. (Ed.). (1981). *The role of the father in child development* (2nd ed.). New York: Wiley.

Lamb, M.E., Thompson, R.A., Gardner, W., Charnov, E.L., & Estes, C. (1984). Security of attachment as assessed in the strange situation: Its study and biological interpretation. *Behavioral and Brain Sciences, 7*, 127–147.

Lewis, M. (1982). The social network systems model: Toward a theory of social development. In T.M. Field, A. Huston, H.C. Quay, L. Troll, & G.E. Finley (Eds.), *Review of human development*. New York: Wiley.

Lipsitt, L.P. (1963). Learning in the first year of life. In L.P. Lipsitt & C.C. Spiker (Eds.), *Advances in child development and behavior* (Vol. 1, pp. 147–195). New York: Academic Press.

Maccoby, E.E., & Martin, J.A. (1983). Socialization in the context of the family: Parent-child interaction. In E.M. Hetherington (Ed.), *Handbook of child psychology* (Vol. 4). New York: Wiley.

Mahler, M., & Pine, F. (1975). *The psychological birth of the infant*. New York: Basic Books.

Nelson, C.A. (1987). The recognition of facial expressions in the first two years of life: Mechanisms of development. *Child Development, 58,* 889–909.

Novak, M.A., & Harlow, H.F. (1975). Social recovery of monkeys isolated for the first year of life. *Developmental Psychology, 11,* 453–465.

Osofsky, J.D. (Ed.). (1979). *Handbook of infant development*. New York: Wiley.

Osofsky, J.D. (Ed.). (1987). *Handbook of infant development* (2nd ed.). New York: Wiley.

Overton, W.F., & Reese, H.W. (1973). Models of development: Methodological implications. In J.R. Neselroade (Ed.), *Life-span developmental psychology: Methodological issues* (pp. 65–86). New York: Academic Press.

Parke, R,D. (1981). *Fathers*. Cambridge, MA: Harvard University Press.

Parke, R,D. (1988). Families in life-span perspective: A multi-level developmental approach. In E.M. Hetherington, R.M. Lerner, & M. Perlmutter (Eds.), *Child development in life-span perspective*. Hillsdale, NJ: Erlbaum.

Parke, R,D. (1989). Social development in infancy: A 25-year perspective. In H.W. Reese (Ed.), *Advances in child development and behavior* (Vol. 21). Orlando, FL: Academic Press.

Parke, R,D., & Ladd, G. (Eds.). (1992). *Family-peer relationships: Modes of linkage*. Hillsdale, NJ: Erlbaum.

Parke, R,D., Power, T.G., & Gottman, J.M. (1979). Conceptualizing and quantifying influence patterns in the family triad. In M.E. Lamb, S.J. Suomi, & G.R. Stephenson (Eds.), *Social interaction analysis: Methodological issues*. Madison, WI: University of Wisconsin Press.

Parke, R.D., & Tinsley, B.J. (1984). Fatherhood: Historical and contemporary perspectives. In K.A. McCluskey & H.W. Reese (Eds.), *Life-span developmental psychology: Historical and generational effects*. New York: Academic Press.

Parke, R.D., & Tinsley, B.J. (1987). Family interaction in infancy. In J.D. Osofsky (Ed.), *Handbook of infant development* (2nd ed., pp. 579–641). New York: Wiley.

Parmalee, A.H., Jr. (1982). Teaching child development and behavioral pediatrics to pediatric trainees. *Society for Research in Child Development Newsletter*, Fall, 1–2.

Pedersen, F.A. (Ed.). (1980). *The father-infant relationship: Observational studies in the family setting*. New York: Praeger Special Studies.

Plomin, R. (1986). *Development, genetics and psychology*. Hillsdale, NJ: Erlbaum.

Plomin, R., & DeFries, J.C. (Eds.). (1985). *Origins of individual differences in infancy: The Colorado adoption project*. Orlando, FL: Academic Press.

Ramey, C.T., MacPhee, D., & Yates, K.O. (1982). Preventing developmental retardation: A general systems model. In L. Bond & J. Joffe (Eds.), *Facilitating infant and early childhood development*. Hanover, NH: University of New England Press.

Reiss, D. (1981). *The family's construction of reality*. Cambridge, MA: Harvard University Press.

Reiss, D., Hetherington, E.M., & Plomin, R. (1990). Non-shared environments in step-families. Unpublished raw data, George Washington University.

Rheingold, H.L. (1956). The modification of social responsiveness in institutional babies. *Monographs of the Society for Research in Child Development*, *21*(63).

Ricciuti, H.N. (1968). Social and emotional behavior in infancy: Some developmental issues and problems. *Merrill-Palmer Quarterly*, *14*, 82–100.

Ricciuti, H.N. (1970). Malnutrition, learning, and intellectual development: Research and remediation. *Psychology and Problems of Society*. Washington, DC: American Psychological Association.

Ricciuti, H.N. (1973). Malnutrition and psychological development. In J. Nurnberger (Ed.), *Biological and environmental determinants of early development* (pp. 63–77). Baltimore, MD: Williams and Wilkins.

Ricciuti, H.N. (1980). Developmental consequences of malnutrition in early childhood. In M. Lewis & L. Rosenblum (Eds.), *The uncommon child: The genesis of development* (Vol. 3). New York: Plenum.

Ricciuti, H.N. (1983). Efectos de los factores ambientales Y nutricionales adversos sobre el desarrolo mental. In *Ambiente, nutricion Y desarrolo mental*, Organizacion Panamericana De La Salud, Publication Cientifica No. 450.

Ricciuti, H.N., & Breitmayer, B. (1988). Observational assessments of infant temperament in the natural setting of the newborn nursery. *Merrill-Palmer Quarterly*, *34*, 281–299.

Ricciuti, H.N., & Thomas, M. (1989, June). Maternal and environmental correlates of quality of infant care in rural families. Paper presented at the American Psychological Society meetings, Alexandria, Virginia.

Rogoff, B. (1990). *Apprenticeship in thinking*. New York: Oxford University Press.

Sackett, G.P. (1968). The persistence of abnormal behavior in monkeys following isolation rearing. In R. Porter (Ed.), *The role of learning in psychotherapy*. London: Churchill.

Sameroff, A.J. (1983). Development systems: Contexts and evolution. In W. Kessen (Ed.), *Handbook of child psychology* (Vol. 1). New York: Wiley.

Sameroff, A.J., & Chandler, M.J. (1975). Reproductive risk and the continuum of caretaking casualty. In F.D. Horowitz, M. Hetherington, S. Scarr-Salapatek, & G. Siegel (Eds.), *Review of child development research* (Vol. 4). Chicago: University of Chicago Press.

Sameroff, A.J., & Emde, R. (Eds.). (1989). *Relationship disturbances in early childhood: A developmental approach*. New York: Basic Books.

Schaffer, H.R. (1984). *The child's entry into a social world*. New York: Academic Press.

Schaffer, H.R., & Emerson, P.E. (1964). The development of social attachments in infancy. *Monographs of the Society for Research in Child Development, 29*(3, Serial No. 94).

Sears, P.R., Maccoby, E.E., & Levin, H. (1957). *Patterns of child rearing*. Evanston, IL: Row Petersen.

Sigel, I.E. (1963). Current research in infant development: Introductory comments. *Merrill-Palmer quarterly, 9*, 81–82.

Sigel, I.E. (1970). Research and teaching of infant development: Introduction. *Merrill-Palmer Quarterly, 16*, 3–6.

Sigel, I.E., & Parke, R.D. (1987). Structural analysis of parent-child research models. *Journal of Applied Developmental Psychology, 8*, 123–137.

Sorce, J.F., Emde, R.N., Klinnert, M.D., & Campos, J.J. (1981, April). Maternal emotional signaling: Its effect on the visual cliff behavior of one-year-olds. Paper presented at the biennial meeting of the Society for Research in Child Development, Boston, Massachusetts.

Spitz, R.A. (1950). Anxiety in infancy: A study of its manifestations in the first year of life. *International Journal of Psychoanalysis, 31*, 138–143.

Sroufe, L.A., & Fleeson, J. (1986). Attachment and the construction of relationships. In W.W. Hartup & Z. Rubin (Eds.), *Relationships and development* (pp. 51–72). Hillsdale, NJ: Erlbaum.

Sroufe, L.A., & Rutter, M. (1984). The domain of developmental psychopathology. *Child Development, 55*, 17–29.

Stern, D.N. (1977). *The first relationship*. Cambridge, MA: Harvard University Press.

Stern, D.N. (1985). *The interpersonal world of the infant*. New York: Basic Books.

Stevenson, H.W., & Siegal, A. (Eds.). (1984). *Child development research and social policy* (Vol. 1). Chicago: University of Chicago Press.

Tinsley, B.J., & Parke, R.D. (1984). The historical and contemporary relationship between developmental psychology and pediatrics: A review and an empirical study. In H.E. Fitzgerald, B.M. Lester, & M.W.

Yogman (Eds.), *Theory and research in behavioral pediatrics* (Vol. 2). New York: Plenum.

Tinsley, B.J., & Parke, R.D. (1987). Grandparents as interactive and social support agents for families with young infants. *International Journal of Aging and Human Development, 25,* 261–279.

Walter, C.A. (1986). *The timing of motherhood.* Lexington, MA: D.C. Heath.

Willis, E.A., & Ricciuti, H.N. (1975). *A good beginning for babies: Guidelines for group care.* Washington, DC: National Association for the Education of Young Children.

Yarrow, L.J. (1961). Maternal deprivation: Toward and empirical and conceptual re-evaluation. *Psychological Bulletin, 58,* 459–490.

Yarrow, L.J. (1964). Separation from parents during early childhood. In M.L. Hoffman & L.W. Hoffman (Eds.), *Review of child development research* (Vol. 1, pp. 89–136). New York: Russell Sage Foundation.

Zajonc, R.B., Murphy, S.T., & Inglehart, M. (1989). Feeling and facial efference: Implications of the vascular theory of emotion. *Psychological Review, 96,* 395–416.

2
Risk and Protective Factors for Parents and Infants[1]

Joy D. Osofsky and Alice Eberhart-Wright

In considering a topic for presentation at this symposium honoring my good friend and colleague, Henry Ricciuti, I tried to choose one that would be consistent with his work over the last 2 decades, the time that I have known him best. In some ways, although he is modest in his temperament and demeanor, I consider Henry a revolutionary with regard to both the quality of his thinking and the programs that he had the courage to develop. He embarked on new ventures and adventures involving infants and their families at times when others confined themselves to the laboratory. In 1969, when I first met Henry, after having joined the faculty at Cornell, I was fascinated with the infant day-care program that he had recently started. Although such programs are not seen as unusual today, in 1969, the majority of researchers, including developmental specialists, questioned the advisability of taking infants out of the home, away from their mothers, and caring for them in a group setting. The infant day-care program that Henry ran in the 1960s and 1970s demonstrated benefits for both the infants and families, and influenced both professionals and parents to consider quality options for alternative care during the early period. At a time when researchers and policymakers were concerned about the effects of out-of-home care for infants on the

[1] The projects described in this chapter were supported by Grant MH–39895 from the National Institute of Mental Health, Center for Prevention Programs and the Institute of Mental Hygiene, New Orleans, Louisiana.

25

developing relationship with the primary caregiver, this program demonstrated that the infants retained the important bond with their mothers while also developing a bond with their day-care caregiver. It should be emphasized that Henry's program had strict requirements for care outside of the home, a number of which cannot be—or are not—followed in most programs today. For example, the mothers were to provide all or most of the care of their infants when they were not in day care, and the group care was restricted to half a day every day. However, the program was important in demonstrating that quality group care for infants can be beneficial in supporting appropriate infant development. Others presenting at this conference have embarked on similar efforts around the same time period with results that substantiate this basic finding.

For me, Henry's program, and the quality of his thinking, were eye-openers. I was always interested in research that had social relevance; prior to my interactions with Henry, most of the infancy work to which I had been exposed had been done in the laboratory with tightly controlled experimental paradigms. In the 1960s, there was relatively little socially relevant applied work being done with infants. The enormous burst in interest and acceptance of observational studies of infancy and the early infant-parent relationship did not occur until the 1970s. In keeping with the theme of this festschrift, and in looking at directions that have been influenced by Henry's important pioneering efforts in the field of infancy, I will provide an overview of some areas of new important research and will then discuss some of our more recent related data.

The Importance of Reciprocity

An extremely important influence on infancy research is the notion of *reciprocity*. Reciprocal relationships between the developing infant and the environment (most often the caregiver) influence both behavioral and affective development. In our work in this area, we have concentrated most recently on affectivity in the early mother-infant relationship. This focus has been used as a way to understand both the infant's use of emotions as a primary means of communication and the degree to which caregivers exert an influence upon their children's overt display, modulation, or control of emotions. In our current work on emotional matching and mismatching in adolescent mothers and their infants, we have observed a changing view of emotional communication and signaling in infancy (Osofsky & Eberhart-Wright, 1988). Previously, emotions were understood as secondary to drives; however, more recently, they have been shown to be important for adaptation in the infant-caregiver relationship (Sameroff & Emde, 1989). Emphasis has been placed on the importance of affective reciprocity for early infant development.

A type of reciprocity is what Stern (1985) describes as *affect attunement*, the ability of parents not only to "read" their infants but also to be resonant with them. The sharing of affectual states is a way of understanding the affective relationship, which is extremely important for the emotional development of the infant. It is the parent's shared affective state that indicates to the infant that a feeling state is understood. If the parent is unable to share the infant's affective state, there is a lack of reciprocity, which we observe fairly often in risk groups. This lack of reciprocity can become problematic if it occurs consistently over time. We will return to this point later.

Another type of reciprocity, which has been described as *emotional availability*, focuses on the caregiver's accessibility and capacity for reading the emotional cues and meeting the emotional needs of the infant. Emde (1980) has suggested that emotional availability may be one of the best barometers of how development is proceeding in early childhood. Under optimal circumstances, we expect to see a range of emotions with a balance of interest and pleasure (positive emotions) between the caregiver and infant. We become concerned about possible problems in the relationship if we observe limited variability and flexibility in the expression of emotions with little positive affect being shown and a sense of there being a dampening of the range of emotions.

Important continuity in experience is provided by affective life. In infancy, emotional signaling between infant and caregiver provides the groundwork for communicating needs, intentions, and satisfactions. Through this process, meaning and motivation are provided, both of which are important in the development of a healthy sense of self. Although self-development occurs within the individual, it is dependent on the presence of the caregiver. How that caregiver communicates and remains emotionally available for the infant influences the developing sense of self. If the caregiver is inconsistently available or out of synchrony with the infant, then it can be expected that there will be problems with important aspects of self-development.

Affect sharing and *affect regulation* are also extremely important in the infant and young child's acquisition of the affective rules inherent to prosocial behaviors, particularly positive affects, empathy, and morality (Emde, 1990). Central to the notion of "good enough mothering" (Bowlby, 1973; Winnicott, 1965) is the ability to be nurturant and emotionally available to the cues and needs of the infant. Positive emotions, which are dependent on nurturance in early relationship experiences, are thought to be extremely important mediators of sociability (Demos, 1989; Emde, 1990). The smile facilitates bonding and attachment, adding to feelings that all is well with the relationship. Infant affects can serve the dual functions of indicating to an observer the present needs of the infant as well as communicating an understanding of positive and negative features of the caregiving relationship. Infant affect may vary with the quality of the caregiving environment. With a more responsive, affectively positive caregiver, greater affective flexibility can be expected in the infant. In contrast, with more negative or inconsistent affective responses from the caregiver, fewer positive and more negative affects can be expected in the infant.

Problems of Reciprocity in Teenage Mothers and Their Infants

As a result of cognitive, maturational, and experiential factors, with increasing age, infants raised with good enough mothering become more capable of resonating with parental affective states. Therefore, it is important to consider risk situations and outcomes for the infant if the mother or caregiver shows little affective resonance or inappropriate and/or inconsistent responses.

During the past several years, first in Topeka, Kansas, and currently in New Orleans, my colleagues and I have been studying teenage mothers, a group frequently considered at risk for problems in adaptive development, and comparing them with primiparous married women. In an earlier paper, we have described patterns of emotional matching and mismatching in adolescent mothers and their infants that relate to developmental risk (Osofsky & Eberhart-Wright, 1988). In the present chapter, we will examine early maternal emotional availability and affect sharing in relation to the development of infant prosocial behaviors and later vulnerability and resiliency.

The subjects on whom the data for this paper are based consisted of 85 mother-infant dyads who were observed when the infants were 13 and 20 months of age. They were part of a larger NIMH-funded longitudinal study in Topeka, Kansas, which began when the young mothers (ages 17 and under) were pregnant and continued until the children were 4.5 years of age. As part of the 13-month assessment, mothers and infants were videotaped during a modified Strange Situation (Ainsworth, Blehar, Waters, & Wall, 1978). During the stranger separation episode, the emotional availability of the mothers was rated on the dimensions of physical and verbal availability with the Emotional Availability scale (Osofsky, Culp, Eberhart-Wright, & Hann, 1989). The presence of positive and negative maternal affect, infant affect, and affect sharing was also rated with this scale. At 20 months, infants were videotaped during a laboratory paradigm designed to measure empathy. They were rated for the presence and degree of both appropriate (empathy, prosocial, exploration, and imitation) and inappropriate (aggression, pleasure, denial, and mixed affect) forms of empathic behavior (Zahn-Waxler & Radke-Yarrow, 1982).

Two of the five types of appropriate empathic behavior were predicted by maternal emotional availability. Prosocial behavior was predicted by greater verbal emotional expressiveness ($r = .23$, $p < .02$), and imitating the distress of the victim was predicted by both verbal emotional expressiveness ($r = .21$, $p < .03$) and attentiveness ($r = .27$, $p < .005$). Out of the four types of inappropriate empathic behavior, aggressive behavior directed toward the victim was found to be predicted by less maternal emotional availability, with greater aggressive behavior associated with less physical availability ($r = -.20$, $p < .05$) and less verbal availability ($r = .21$, $p < .05$).

We next investigated the relationships between 13-month measures of affect sharing and 20-month measures of empathic behavior. Three of the five indices of appropriate empathic behavior were associated with measures of affect sharing. Empathic behavior at 20 months was associated with fewer instances of earlier nonshared child negative affect ($r = -.27$, $p < .006$). Child prosocial behavior was inversely related to the display of no affect ($r = -.22$, $p < .05$) and positively associated with instances of positive affect sharing ($r = .26$, $p < .01$) and nonshared child positive affect ($r = .18$, $p < .01$). Showing mastery of the situation (i.e., acting as caregiver) was associated with both positive affect sharing ($r = .21$, $p < .05$) and mixed questionable affect exchanges ($r = .25$, $p < .01$). Similarly, exploration of the situation (i.e., asking questions) was associated with previous mixed questionable affect exchanges ($r = .18$, $p < .05$). Two of the four indices of inappropriate empathic behavior were related to earlier measures of affect sharing, with both pleasure and affect confusion associated with nonshared maternal positive affect ($r = .22$, $p < .02$, and $r = .19$, $p < .05$, respectively).

Overall, the findings for 13- and 20-month-old infants and their young mothers showed that greater emotional availability and positive affect sharing were associated with appropriate empathic responses by the infant at 20 months. Negative affect sharing and nonsharing by the mother were associated with fewer empathic responses and those that were inappropriate. These results support the notion that early responsiveness to infant emotional signals and the sharing of positive affect may influence the later development of empathy and prosocial behaviors. Based on this theoretical and empirical information, we have concerns about the outcomes for the infant if the mother or caregiver shows little affective resonance or inappropriate and/or inconsistent responses, which occur frequently with young mothers and infants. With such inappropriate or mixed affect exchanges, the child may react with a number of options that may then become a pattern within the relationship. For example, the child may act the same way again and again in order to elicit a response from the mother, or the child may explore less or take less initiative because such behaviors tend to result in negative responses from the mothers. In addition, the child may develop an inaccurate or distorted sense of self as a result of the inappropriate or mixed-affect exchanges. If the infant's affective state is consistently misinterpreted, then he or she may begin to behave in inappropriate ways both with mother and others. The infant has learned what to expect in the exchange. It is possible to speculate that each type of inappropriate affective exchange will result in a distinctive type of experience for the infant. If such experiences occur repeatedly in the infant-mother system, then they may begin to influence the child's developing sense of self.

Emde (1990) has emphasized the importance of positive affect sharing in the relationship. Studying normative samples, he has described an interesting phenomenon that occurs toward the end of the first year of life, one in which considerable individual dif-

ferences are apparent. Children of this age tend to look to a significant other and to share positive affect, for example, sharing
a smile during exploration or after an accomplishment. Positive
affect sharing is a sensitive indicator that all is well with development and with the relationship. When we have carried out
comparable studies with young mothers and infants, we have
observed less positive and more negative affect than in Emde's
normative group. Further, we have observed a great deal of nonsharing of affects in the relationship. For example, the infant
may express an affective response to which the mother will not
respond, and there will not be reciprocity. We feel that such interactions place the infant or young child at risk for current and
later problems in development and in his or her developing relationships. Further, there is some evidence that positive affective
inclinations may be associated with individuals who "steel" or
"buffer" themselves during times of stress. The implications for
gaining better understanding of resiliency and invulnerability,
especially in risk groups, are important.

Evidence for Protective Factors

In our past and ongoing studies of young mothers and their infants,
we are continually impressed with the problems in reciprocity that
seem to be common in these mother-child relationships. Many of
the young mothers and infants exhibit problems for a variety of
reasons, including the mother's youthful age and her own developmental concerns and issues. In addition, they are linked to
continuing generations of poverty; limited educational resources
and the ability to utilize them; few successful role models in the
immediate environment; and, for all of the above reasons, frequent
disorganization within the immediate family and broader supportive community. Despite all of these problems, which seem for
many to be part of being a young mother, there are some mothers
and infants who do well—or at least do much better than might be
expected considering their circumstances and opportunities. Based
on these successes, we are studying factors that lead to relative
invulnerability or resiliency for young mothers and children.

Before discussing the specific "protective" factors that we have
observed in young mothers and their children, and describing
several of the cases, it may be helpful to consider briefly some of
the characteristics that others have identified in the resilient or

invulnerable child. Garmezy (1983) and Garmezy, Masten, and Tellegen (1984), in a series of studies with families of poverty, have isolated a number of factors that are associated with increased resistance to stress for children. These include an ability to relate positively to peers, adequate intelligence, and some significant support available in the environment. Other investigators (Felsman & Valliant, 1987) have suggested that children who are resilient seem to be able to use flexible coping strategies in overcoming adversity. They are more able to be reflective rather than impulsive in solving problems (Kagan, Rosman, Day, Albert, & Phillips, 1964). Still others have indicated that resilient children are able to use more goal-oriented strategies in planning means for overcoming problems rather than feeling hopeless. They are also able to plan ahead rather than just acting on the moment. Of particular significance, more resilient children who live in a socially disorganized environment show an increased capacity for comforting and soothing themselves rather than having to depend upon others for comfort (Cohler, 1987).

Furstenberg, Brooks-Gunn, and Morgan (1987), in their 17-year follow-up of a sample of teenage mothers and their children in Baltimore found several factors to be extremely important for more successful outcomes. The young mothers' being able to continue with educational goals affected outcomes for both them and their children in terms of their feelings about themselves and their economic opportunities. The mothers' limiting their fertility was a second factor that positively influenced outcomes. A third major influence that seemed to impact greatly on their economic situation was whether they were married and stayed married before or after the birth of their child, which provided a steady income to allow the family to be self-supporting. Furstenberg et al. pointed out, however, that this latter factor may have played a more significant role for a cohort growing up in the 1960s than it would today. In terms of outcomes for the children of teenage mothers, "no single model described the impact of maternal career contingencies on the course of the children's development" (p. 145). However, several factors were predictive of poor outcomes, including welfare dependency; high fertility; and, at different developmental periods, marital status and family support. They concluded in terms of implications for public policy that part of the handicap of being a teenage mother may come from a widespread perception that failure is inevitable. Yet many of the young mothers that they studied 17 years later were doing better than expected and much better than they had been doing for the first 5 years after they had the child.

In our study of teenage mothers in Topeka, Kansas, we have also been impressed with the growing strength of young mothers over time. Although we have followed them for less time (4.5 years), we have observed many positive changes in some mothers during that time period both in terms of their own life structure and their ability to relate positively to their children. The Furstenberg et al. (1987) data have shown that academic interests and abilities seem to play an important role in that those adolescents who were educationally ambitious and at grade level when they became pregnant were the most likely to avoid later economic dependency and excess fertility. In the latest report of our longitudinal study (Osofsky, Ware, Culp, & Eberhart-Wright, 1989), we have found that self-esteem seems to be an important factor affecting positive outcomes 3 to 4 years later for both teenage mothers and their children. Further, whether the young mothers have been able to obtain a general equivalency diploma (GED) and a job after having a baby at a young age also seems to impact, to a significant extent, outcomes in their lives and those of their children.

For this group of teenage mothers (age 17 and under) and their children, we have been attempting to go further in identifying possible protective factors in both the mothers and children. Our results to date have been consistent with the findings of other studies with risk populations. For child factors, we have been able to identify the following: the child's inherent intelligence; ability to charm others rather than attack; ability to use available resources whatever they might be; extended family or other supports to relieve negative experiences; ability to adjust to change (adaptability); zest for living; factors that compensate for weaknesses; ability to use symbolic play to relieve negative factors; and ability to cooperate with adults despite the child's own wishes. Maternal factors that appear protective for the children include: the mother's always being there emotionally (even if she is negative or inconsistent); protection from mother's crises; the mother's ability to put her own life together and work on bettering herself; her ability to use intervention; her having goals for her life; and her ability to express negatives in her life and be positive with her child.

In reviewing 59 mother-child dyads in our young mother population who have been followed until the children were 4.5 years of age, we have been impressed by the great variability and number of complex patterns that have developed since the children were born. Twenty-two of the cases show clear signs of resiliency and important protective factors in either the mother, child, or dyad. Three of these cases have been selected to illustrate some of the protective factors involved. Case 1 focuses on the mother and the positive factors that she uses to protect her child from her own adolescent chaos. Case 2 presents a child who develops impressive resiliency with little support from consistent caregivers. Case 3 describes reciprocal protective factors in a mother and child whose physical survival depended on unusual resiliency.

Case 1: Danielle and Jennifer

Danielle was 17 when she gave birth to tiny Jennifer. Danielle had smoked throughout her pregnancy, which may have affected Jennifer's relatively low birth weight. Nonetheless, Danielle seemed attached to her baby, nursed her, and took her home to an intact family unit. Like most children of the teenage mother population, Jennifer was an unplanned child whose mother was not married and had not finished school when Jennifer was conceived.

The protective factors that enabled Jennifer to excel at 4.5 years were already evident from early on in the relationship. When she learned that she was expecting a baby, Danielle completed work for her GED and married the father of her child, showing her capacity to have goals and plan ahead. She enlisted the support of her parents and was able to work through their difficult negative reaction to her pregnancy. During our feeding observation in the hospital following delivery, Danielle was unusually animated with her baby, who was temperamentally responsive to her mother's interactions.

For the next few years, Danielle struggled. Her husband had an alcohol problem and became abusive. After trying to make the marriage work by seeking marriage counseling, Danielle gave up. Even when the marriage was most chaotic, Danielle protected Jennifer. After she and her husband were separated, Danielle would not allow Jennifer to go with him if he had been drinking. Although Danielle sometimes struggled with depression and self-esteem problems, she was always emotionally available to Jennifer, responding to her in an animated manner even when her own life was in turmoil. As Jennifer experienced many moves, a succession of possible new father figures, and even a bout of a serious illness that required hospitalization, she could count on her mother being there to protect her. In addition, her grandparents were always there to nurture both of them, allowing them to move into their house periodically for a short time.

Not only did Danielle protect Jennifer from the difficulties in her own life, but she also encouraged Jennifer's innate strengths—her intelligence and her strong will. Danielle loved to teach Jennifer and bought her toys designed to challenge her next stage of development. Unlike many young mothers, she talked to her consistently and enjoyed listening and responding to Jennifer's conversational efforts as she acquired language. Behavior that could have been construed as defiance by some parents was interpreted as independence and a strong will by Danielle, who delighted in pointing it out to the evaluators.

Consequently, at 4.5 years, Jennifer was a child who tested in the superior range on intelligence tests, related very well to adults, and drew with strong black lines an age-appropriate self-portrait that filled the page, indicative of healthy self-esteem.

Protective factors in this case focus on the mother:

1. Consistent emotional availability.
2. Ability to utilize support from the outside.
3. Goals (GED and job).
4. Shielding the child from parental crises.
5. Acknowledging and working on areas of difficulty in her own life.
6. An increasing ability to make choices based on thought rather than emotion, showing an ability to delay gratification.
7. An ability to attune herself to the child's changing needs and provide what was needed at each developmental stage.
8. Seeing parenting as a priority in life.

The child's protective factors included her innate intelligence and physical attractiveness, which in combination with her mother's protectiveness enabled her to be unusually successful in all of the areas that were assessed when she was 54 months of age.

Case 2: Anita and Daniel

Daniel's struggles began the day he was born. As we watched his 17-year-old mother, Anita, feed him in the hospital, we noted that she left the bottle hanging in his mouth while she talked on the phone. In no uncertain terms, she told him that he would have to get used to her since they would be together at least 18 years. Already Daniel was developing the charm that would help him survive. Notes from the Brazelton newborn assessment indicated that Daniel was a wonderful cuddler and worked hard to respond to the examiner even when he was sleepy. He was the kind of baby anyone would want to take home—cuddly, responsive, and attractive, with his dark curly hair and long eyelashes framing big expressive eyes. Weighing over 8 pounds, he was physically ready to take on the world.

Daniel needed to be ready for the world. For the next 4.5 years, we kept track of his whereabouts through police reports in the newspaper. His numerous homes were repeatedly burglarized, and his mother was arrested periodically for drug dealing. Father figures came and went, and Anita's chaotic family mainly interacted through fighting. Although Daniel developed new skills with each evaluation, Anita seemed stuck—no high school diploma or GED, no job, no stable relationships, no goals. Anita was totally unaware of what good parenting entailed. She fed Daniel before our cameras by sticking him under the rocking chair with a bottle, teased and slapped him, and was mostly emotionally unavailable. For a period of about 6 months before and after his first birthday, Daniel was in foster care. At the 20-month evaluation, Daniel showed insecure-avoidant behavior during the strange situation. Daniel's performances at 44 and 54 months amazed us. Although scoring low on standardized tests, he worked hard, had a long attention span, and passed selected items at the 5- and 6-year-old levels on the Stanford-Binet intelligence scale. He solved story problems with a mixture of aggressive and prosocial solutions but showed empathy and caring. When given time to develop his own scripts, he had the mother and father dolls go to work.

Frequently coming to evaluations barefoot and dirty, Daniel's play was organized and appropriate. Although his speech was hard to understand, he communicated well through repetition, gestures, and delightful facial animation. At 4.5 years, he demanded fairness from his mother in the bowling game, insisted on pursuing his own interests despite pressure from her to do what she wanted, and solicited support from the new father figure when his mother slapped him. Instead of becoming angry and aggressive in frustrating situations, he cried beseechingly, which tapped strong maternal instincts in his immature mother. Figure drawings of father, mother, and self depicted bizarre abstract figures for parents and an intact self. At 4.5 years, Daniel had a zest for living that could be considered surprising in light of his life experiences.

Protective factors for the child included the following:

1. A healthy start (in this case enabling Daniel to bounce back from severe asthma attacks).
2. Physical attractiveness that lured outside adults into providing positive attention.
3. A social nature apparent from birth.
4. The development of relational skills that elicited support rather than punishment.
5. A drive to enjoy life regardless of circumstances.
6. An ability to adapt to change rapidly and make the best of new situations.
7. A long attention span and interest in learning.
8. Role reversal so that the emphasis was no attunement to mother rather than vice versa.
9. An ability to care for and nurture himself.
10. An ability to use symbolic play to master difficult life situations and create a different type of life.

Case 3: Patty and Erin

At 17, Patty gave birth prematurely to Erin, who was so tiny that she required hospitalization for several months. The initial social work assessment described Patty as being immature and depressed. At the hospital, the nursing staff worried that they could not count on Patty to come for feedings when she said she would. When we observed Patty feeding Erin, we have impressed with how much Erin looked at Patty.

For the next 4.5 years, the road was rough for both Patty and Erin. Erin required repeated hospitalizations for various surgical procedures as well as failure to thrive. When we saw her for an evaluation at 8 months, she looked so sickly and weak that we were concerned about her ability to survive much longer. Patty made poor choices in her initial relationships, which echoed her life growing up in a dysfunctional family. The home visitor termination note at 30 months indicated that Patty had frequently failed appointments and had made mixed use of intervention. The home visitor considered her at high risk for further problems.

As we watched Patty and Erin grow, we noted that Erin was an even-tempered, responsive child who capitalized on whatever Patty had to offer. Patty was inconsistently emotionally available, sometimes drifting off into her own thoughts and forgetting Erin. Occasionally, she referred to Erin as a brat but did so in a positive tone of voice.

At the 54-month evaluation, we were impressed at the growth that both Erin and Patty had made. Although Erin was not an attractive child, she compensated by being charming with adults. Her mother dressed her in cute clothes and always made sure she was clean, with carefully combed long hair. Erin had always scored low on intelligence tests but compensated by having a long attention span and cooperating with all performance demands. She was able to pass word definitions at the 5-year level, reflecting a good use of language. Script play at 44 months depicted a rich use of symbolic play and all prosocial solutions to problems.

By 54 months after Erin's birth, Patty was married to a man who had a good job and supported the family well. Although Patty still struggled with feelings of low self-esteem, she was no longer significantly depressed. She was able to talk about the things she liked and did not like about parenting, and had goals to finish school and obtain further training. She had enrolled Erin in a good intervention preschool to help her with her developmental delays. She talked about emotional support from her husband, mother, and church.

The inconsistent pattern of emotional availability that we had observed from birth persisted. Patty still retreated into her own world before our cameras. The striking development was Erin's understanding and patience with that phenomenon. When her mother did not respond to her, she waited patiently, neither retreating nor demanding—simply giving time to her mother to tune in to her again. Then Patty showed us the "good enough mothering" pattern that resulted in Erin's survival—helping, talking, and simply always being there.

Protective factors for the child included the following:

1. A drive to grow and develop rather than bailing out during difficult times.
2. Compensating factors for weaknesses (i.e., charm instead of beauty, symbolic richness instead of intellect, socioemotional health instead of physical health, perseverance with learning rather than ease of learning).
3. The acceptance of positive support systems over time.
4. The availability and utilization of medical and educational community resources at critical times.

Protective factors for the dyad included the following:

1. The ability to adapt to one another's needs and unique characteristics.
2. Educational goals for both mother and child.

Discussion

Focusing on risk and protective factors in adolescent mothers and their infants is unlike our usual concerns with vulnerability and resiliency. In this case, we have the unique opportunity to study two immature individuals—actually two children—struggling to survive, develop, and grow. Therefore, we must consider protective factors for the infants and children, those for the young mother, and the broader family and community factors that may have an impact on the dyad. As these two individuals—the mother and child—interact, more risk may be created for the dyad.

Earlier in the paper, we noted problems in reciprocity that are common in adolescent mother-child relationships. The mother's youthful age and her own developmental conflicts contribute to these problems. Further, opportunities to observe and learn how to interact in a positive reciprocal manner may be hampered due to disorganization in the environment and the continual assaults related to the mother's age and, frequently, a life of poverty. Emotional availability and affect attunement occur much less often for young mothers than for commonly accepted normative groups. One must depend on what Fraiberg (1975) and, more recently, Emde (1990) refer to as the positive "developmental thrust" of the infant and child that moves both the child and the dyad forward in development. Thus, the resiliency of the first mother-child pair discussed above was due to both the inherent competency of the youngster and the mother's ability to continue to protect her despite her own, at times, chaotic environment. For the second dyad, the child's positive developmental thrust and zest for life allowed him to survive despite his mother's inadequacy as a parent. The third dyad was at particular risk due to the medical condition and continuing physical problems of the child. Although the mother was inconsistent in her emotional availability, the child was able to compensate for her physical weakness, and they were able to adapt together to their special needs. Together, this mother and child appeared to be more resilient than many pairs that we have observed.

Garmezy (1983) and Rutter (1979) have identified important distinguishing features in either the individual child, parent, or environment that contribute to invulnerability or resiliency. We have identified similar factors in either the children or young mothers that seem to protect some of the children of teenage mothers as well as the young mothers themselves. For the children, we have identified inherent strengths, including intelligence, positive temperamental characteristics, and ability to cooperate and nurture oneself to some extent. For the mothers, emotional availability seems to be extremely important, even if it is variable. The mother's ability to use available community resources appears to make a difference, as does her motivation and capacity to have goals and plans for her life. We have found that the mother's ability to be aware of and express the negatives in her life and, at the same time, be positive with her child seems to make a difference for both her and her child.

The study of teenage mothers and their infants and children broadens our perspective on risk and protective factors in development. Here, we have two at-risk individuals, both of whom need protective factors to survive. They are both vulnerable, yet in some cases they show both individual and dyadic resiliency. Our task is to identify what it is in these young mothers and infants that leads to resiliency and success. How can we enhance the reciprocity in their relationship and help the mothers become more emotionally available to their infants? All of these questions are extremely important with regard to efforts to develop more effective preventive intervention strategies.

References

Ainsworth, M.D.S., Blehar, M., Waters, E., & Wall, S. (1978). *Patterns of attachment.* Hillsdale, NJ: Erlbaum.

Bowlby, J. (1973). *Attachment and loss* (Vol. 2). New York: Basic Books.

Cohler, B. (1987). Adversity, resilience, and the study of lives. In E.J. Anthony & B. Cohler (Eds.), *The Invulnerable Child* (pp. 363–424). New York: The Guilford Press.

Demos, E.V. (1989). Resiliency in infancy. In T.F. Dugan & R. Coles (Eds.), *The child in our times* (pp. 3–22). New York: Brunner/Mazel.

Emde, R.N. (1980). Emotional availability: A reciprocal reward system for infants and parents with implications for prevention of psychosocial disorders. In P.M. Taylor (Ed.), *Parent-infant relationships* (pp. 87–115). Orlando, FL: Grune & Stratton.

Emde, R.N. (1990). Lessons from infancy: New beginnings in a changing world and a morality for health. *Infact Mental Health Journal, 11*, 196–212.

Felsman, J.K., & Valliant, G.E. (1987). Resilient children as adults: A 40-year study. In E.J. Anthony & B.J. Cohler (Eds.), *The Invulnerable Child* (pp. 289–314). New York: The Guilford Press.

Fraiberg, S., Adelson, E., & Shapiro, V. (1975). Ghosts in the nursery: A psychoanalytic approach to the problems of impaired infant-mother relationships. *Journal of the American Academy of Child Psychiatry, 14,* 387–421.

Furstenberg, F.F., Jr., Brooks-Gunn, J., & Morgan, S.P. (1987). *Adolescent mothers in later life.* New York: Cambridge University Press.

Garmezy, N. (1983). Stressors of childhood. In M. Rutter & N. Garmezy (Eds.), *Stress, coping, and development in children* (pp. 43–84). New York: McGraw-Hill.

Garmezy, N., Masten, A.S., & Tellegen, A. (1984). The study of stress and competence in children: A building block for developmental psychopathology. *Child Development, 55,* 97–111.

Kagan, J., Rosman, B.L., Day, D., Albert, J., & Phillips, W. (1964). Information processing in the child: Significance of analytic and reflective attitudes. *Psychological Monographs, 78*(1, Whole No. 578).

Osofsky, J.D., & Eberhart-Wright, A. (1988). Affective exchanges between high risk mothers and infants. *International Journal of Psychoanalysis, 69,* 221–231.

Osofsky, J.D., Culp, A.M., & Eberhart-Wright, A. & Hann, D.M. (1989). *Final Report for Kenworthy-Swift Foundation.* The Menninger Clinic, Topeka, and Louisiana State University Medical Center, New Orleans.

Rutter, M. (1979). Protective factors in children's responses to stress and disadvantage. In M.W. Kent & J.D. Rolf (Eds.), *Primary prevention of psychopathology, Vol. 3: Social competence in children* (pp. 49–74). Hanover, NH: University Press of New England.

Sameroff, A., & Emde, R.N. (Eds.). (1989). *Relationship Disturbances in early childhood.* New York: Basic Books.

Stern, D. (1985). *The interpersonal world of the infant.* New York: Basic.

Winnicott, D. (1965). *The maturational processes and the facilitating environment.* New York: International Universities Press.

Zahn-Waxler, C., & Radke-Yarrow, M. (1982). The development of altruism: Alternative research strategies. In N. Eisenberg (Ed.), *The Development of Prosocial Behavior* (pp. 109–137). New York: Academic Press.

3

Long-Term Developmental Consequences of Intrauterine and Postnatal Growth Retardation in Rural Guatemala

Ernesto Pollitt, Kathleen Gorman,
and Elizabeth Metallinos-Katsaras

Introduction

Knowledge on the developmental consequences of low birth weight (LBW) infants is derived primarily from research in developed countries such as the United States and Great Britain (Friedman & Sigman, 1981; Vietze & Vaughan, 1988). In that context it is now recognized that except for extreme cases, LBW is not a sufficient cause for developmental deviation. In fact, the final developmental outcome of LBW infants is often determined by the nature of the social environment to which the LBW child is exposed after birth rather than by the child's intrauterine history (Hack & Breslau, 1988; Sameroff & Chandler, 1975; Werner & Smith, 1977). The social environment acts as either a buffer against the potential effects of the prenatal trauma or as a remedial agent that corrects a deviation that may be apparent in early life (Ricciuti, 1989).

What is much less known is what happens with LBW children in developing countries. In particular, there is a scarcity of information on the developmental trajectory of LBW infants born in social settings where poverty coexists with a high incidence of infectious diseases and macro- and micronutrient deficiencies (Mata, 1978). In those situations, intrauterine history may be a powerful determinant of the infant's developmental trajectory because the social environment may lack the preventative or remedial properties present in the social environments in developed countries.

In an attempt to fill in the gap in the available information, this chapter reports on the long-term developmental outcomes of children with a history of intrauterine growth retardation (IUGR) born into a nutritionally at-risk population in rural Guatemala. In particular, the concern is with the functional performance of adolescents whose body size and proportions at birth and whose body size at 1 year of life suggested different nutritional histories in utero and early postnatal life.

Developmental Risk and Intrauterine Growth Retardation (IUGR)

Low birth weight is a broad diagnostic category that includes conditions of different pathogenicity and developmental risk. A finer degree of differentiation between the clinical groups that fit into such a category has proven valuable in terms of both the definitions of causality and prognosis. Recent studies on IUGR point to the developmental and clinical importance of distinguishing between growth-retarded infants with and without anthropometric symmetry at birth (i.e., symmetry as defined by ponderal index [PI: weight/height^3]). Proportional (Type I, or symmetrical: adequate ponderal index [API]) and disproportional (Type II, or asymmetrical: low ponderal index [LPI]) IUGR are assumed to have different pathogenicity. Symmetrical IUGR is most prevalent in developing countries and is believed to be the result of nutritional deficiencies throughout most or all of pregnancy (Lin & Evans, 1984; Ounsted, Moar, & Scott, 1986; Villar & Belizan, 1982). On the other hand, asymmetrical IUGR is more likely to be observed in industrialized countries and is associated with deviant intrauterine growth primarily during the last trimester of pregnancy. Differences in the postnatal growth and developmental trajectories of symmetrical and asymmetrical IUGR infants are expected.

Haas, Balcazar, and Caulfield (1987) showed that dysmorphic or asymmetrical growth-retarded infants in Mexico and Bolivia had higher mortality rates than symmetrical IUGR and normal infants. Asymmetrical infants had 2.9 to 5.7 times the mortality rate of the full-term appropriate-weight infants. Symmetrically growth-retarded infants had, in turn, nearly twice the mortality rate of the full-term appropriate-weight infants. On the other hand, Villar and Belizan (1982) reported that IUGR infants with symmetrical body proportions tend to remain small, whereas IUGR infants with asymmetrical body proportions more frequently catch up with normal birth weight infants (Villar & Belizan, 1982; Villar, Smeriglio, Martorell, Brown, & Klein, 1984).

The notions of differential risk and nutritional history in utero between symmetrical and asymmetrical infants are also derived from experiments with supplementary feeding. Mueller and Pollitt (1984) observed in Taiwan that the effects of an energy protein supplement among pregnant women varied according to the anthropometric characteristics of the conceptus. In utero, infants at risk of dysmorphic growth (i.e., asymmetric IUGR) benefited the most from maternal supplementation, as suggested by a comparatively higher birth weight.

Although the data from Guatemala suggest that asymmetrical infants are better-off, the data from Mexico and Bolivia suggest the converse. A solution to this apparent contradiction is found in the timing at which risk was assessed. Asymmetrical IUGR infants were found to be at a higher risk immediately after birth, and this is not surprising given that the time of their insult is likely to have occurred immediately before—that is, in the last trimester of pregnancy. Symmetrical infants who experienced deficiencies in the maternal supply of nutrients throughout gestation suffer a reduction in both cell division and cell growth. This would explain their body growth retardation at 36 months.

Figure 3.1 is illustrative. It presents the intrauterine changes in growth velocity for body size and body growth (Belizan & Villar, 1988). The peak of growth velocity for body size occurs at about the 20th week of gestation, whereas that of body weight occurs at the 33rd week. Accordingly, the low weight for size in a newborn with asymmetrical body proportions points to a stress in the last trimester of pregnancy. Therefore, mortality and morbidity risk is likely to be high immediately after birth. On the other hand, an infant with symmetrical dimensions suggests that stress was present throughout pregnancy and affected both size and weight.

Studies on the long-term developmental or behavioral consequences of IUGR have generally failed to classify subjects according to body proportions at birth, and consequently, the results appear contradictory. For example, Westwood, Kramer, Munz, Lovett, and Watters (1983) did not find differences in cognitive development among adolescents who were born with and without IUGR, whereas Hill et al. (1984) and Rantakallio (1985) reported that IUGR affected school performance and intelligence test scores

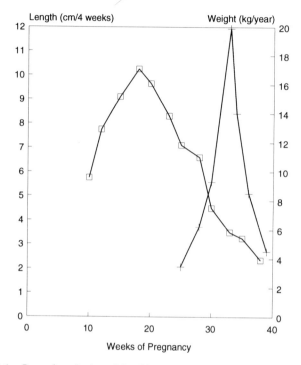

FIGURE 3.1. Growth velocity of fetal length and weight during the prenatal period. Adapted from Belizan and Villar (1988) with permission.

of adolescents. In one of the very few studies comparing symmetrical and asymmetrical IUGR infants in a developing country, Villar and Belizan (1982) found that at 3 years of age, symmetrical IUGR infants scored lower than asymmetrical IUGR infants on discrimination learning tasks, memory, and vocabulary tests. The asymmetrical infants, on the other hand, performed as well as the controls in all but one (i.e., digit span) of the cognitive tests.

Postnatal Growth

Because postnatal malnutrition is often highly prevalent, it is to be expected that in developing countries the developmental trajectory of LBW infants will depend heavily on the nature of the physical and biological environment to which they are exposed after birth. Within such a framework it could be assumed that the developmental risk of infants whose intrauterine growth retardation is secondary to nutritional deficiencies is likely to differ as a function of the extent to which postnatal nutritional needs are met.

Linear growth retardation is pronounced in low-income children from developing countries, particularly during the first 2 years of postnatal life (Martorell & Habicht, 1986). A common observation is that growth in length during the first 3 to 6 months of life falls on or close to the 50th percentile of the reference standards of Western societies; however, by 12 to 24 months of life the infants fall below the 5th percentile. This shift results in a remarkable change in the contour of the growth curve and a swift decline of growth velocity. Numerous reasons exist for this growth change, but generally they involve an intake of macro- (e.g., calories) and micronutrients (e.g., iron) below physiological requirements, and high rates of infection, particularly diarrheal diseases.

Postnatal macro- and micronutrient requirements increase during periods of accelerated physical growth. Illustrative is the case of iron; the requirements estimated by mg/kg are particularly high during the first 6 to 12 months, and the prevalence of iron deficiency within a population (e.g., the United States) is highest among infants (Pilch & Senti, 1984). Periods of accelerated growth, either prenatally or postnatally, accentuate the vulnerability of the organism to noxious agents or nutritional deficiencies. Again in connection with iron, it has been postulated that the developmental risk associated with iron deficiency anemia is particularly high in infancy (Lozoff, 1989). Thus, in comparison to other developmental periods in early and later childhood, the infant is not only more likely to become nutritionally deficient but is also more vulnerable to biological insults.

Through possibly different pathways, morbidity, low energy intake, and iron and zinc deficiencies dalay postnatal linear growth (Mata, 1978). Each of these conditions has also been associated with either central nervous system dysfunction or developmental delays in infancy as indicated by low developmental scale scores (Halas, 1983; Joos & Pollitt, 1984; Lozoff, 1989; Pollitt, 1983; Ricciuti, 1981b; Thomson & Pollitt, 1977). Thus a positive covariation between growth retardation and developmental delay in infancy is expected, particularly in populations where malnutrition is endemic.

Retarded body growth during the first 12 to 24 months of postnatal life, associated with severe protein energy malnutrition

(PEM), has been correlated with school failure as indicated by repetition of grades, low achievement test scores, and comparatively poor performance on IQ tests (Pollitt, 1988). To the extent of our knowledge, there are no data on growth retardation in infancy associated with mild-to-moderate PEM and performance in primary schooling. One possible exception is the study of malnourished infants in Korea who were adopted by American families and brought to the United States, thereafter living under middle-class conditions. The school performance of these Korean children was comparable to that of an average public school child (Winick & Meyer, 1975).

In summary, the available evidence suggests that IUGR, symmetrical body proportions at birth, and growth retardation during the first 12 to 24 months of life are risk factors likely to alter the long-term developmental trajectory of children from a normal course. Although the evidence available is not sufficient to establish specific hypotheses regarding developmental effects of the interactions between these factors, there is theoretical justification to assume that the effects will be more clearly apparent when two or more of these factors are present. On the basis of these considerations, this study was designed to test the long-term independent and interactive effects of IUGR, body proportions, and retarded physical growth at 12 months.

Methods

The longitudinal study on which the following analysis is based was carried out from 1969 to 1989 in four rural ladino (non-Indian) villages in the Department of E1 Progreso in eastern Guatemala by both the Institute of Nutrition of Central America and Panama and a consortium of universities. The objective of the original study was to assess the functional consequences of early supplementary feeding among infants and children. The primary hypothesis tested in that study was that nutrition affects mental development (Townsend et al., 1982) and physical growth of preschool-aged children (Martorell, Delgado, Valverde, & Klein, 1981). This hypothesis is not directly related to the present purposes; therefore, the issue of supplementation is not discussed further. The study included two distinct periods of data collection on the same subjects. One followed a longitudinal format spanning from 1969 to 1977 and included complete schooling records collected in 1988;

the other was cross-sectional and was restricted to 1988 and 1989. The study population was composed of all the residents (3,500 inhabitants according to a 1975 census) of the four villages.

The Villages

The following description of the four villages is rooted in three socioeconomic surveys conducted in 1967, 1974, and 1987. All four villages are located in a dry, mountainous area northeast of Guatemala City. Their elevation ranges from 275 to 1,250 meters above sea level. The lowest and highest temperatures are from about 14 to 38 degrees centigrade. Two major crops in each village are corn and beans; in addition, tomatoes, sorghum, and yucca are important crops in some of the villages.

HOUSING

The typical house in three of the four villages has one to two rooms with adobe walls, dirt floors, and a tile or metal roof. In the remaining village, where the climate is warmest, most houses have thatched roofs, and the walls are made of reeds and mud. In 1967, almost all houses had dirt floors, but by 1987 roughly one third of the houses in three of the villages and two thirds in the fourth village had cement floors. The kitchen is usually either a separate room or located in a separate area just outside the house. Most people own their homes, as well as at least some of the land around their homes.

Electricity was not available in any of the villages in 1967. By 1974, one village had electricity, to which about half of the families in this village had access. By 1987, two thirds to three fourths of all families in the four villages had electricity in their homes.

Related to the availability of electricity are data on availability of appliances. In 1967, about one third of the families had radios; by 1987 half or more (two thirds in one village) owned radios. In 1987, only a few (<5%) owned a record player, refrigerator, or bicycle, whereas between 15 and 30% owned televisions.

In 1967, there were virtually no households with any prescribed means of feces disposal. By 1974, about 10% of the households in all the villages except one had rudimentary septic tanks for waste disposal; in the one exception about 5% had septic tanks and 17% had latrines. By 1987, roughly one half to two thirds of the families in each village had some means of sanitation at their homes. In general, water systems and methods of human waste disposal are still not well developed.

OCCUPATION

The primary means of income for most villagers is agricultural production. Almost all are tenant farmers or small landowners. No one in any of the villages reported being a large landholder, and very few reported being merchants. Agricultural wage labor is not a principal occupation except in one village, where basket weaving from palm leaves is common. The percentage of men who report working in skilled trades has increased from very few in 1967 to between 20 and 50% in 1987. Very few women report having an occupation in any of the villages except one, where women earn money independently through basket weaving.

LITERACY AND SCHOOLING

The percentage of mothers reporting to be at least partially literate in each village ranged from 25 to 40% in 1967 and from 58 to 63% in 1987. The range of literacy of fathers increased from between 38 and 60% in 1967 to between 61 and 76% in 1987. Figures 3.2 and 3.3 present the changes in mothers' and fathers' literacy over time, respectively. By 1987, in at least three of the villages, the gap between the literacy rates for women and men had been greatly

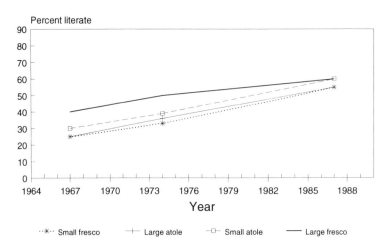

FIGURE 3.2. Changes in literacy of mothers by village and year.

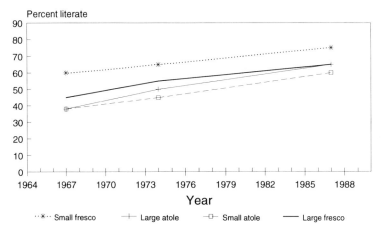

FIGURE 3.3. Changes in literacy of fathers by village and year.

reduced. Literacy has improved over the years at remarkably similar rates in all the villages, except in one village where initial rates were higher.

DEMOGRAPHY

The population in each village has approximately doubled since 1967, with growth rates for the villages appearing to be similar across villages. Figure 3.4 presents the change from 1967 to 1987 in the number of families in each village graphically, whereas Figure

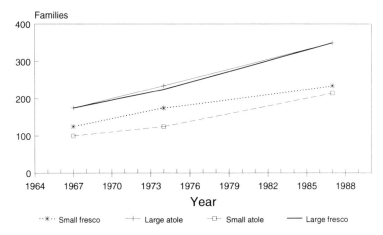

FIGURE 3.4. Change in number of families by village and year.

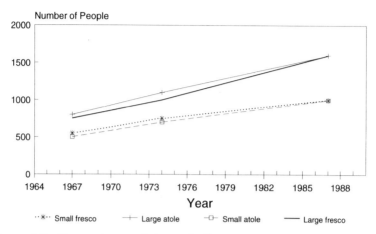

FIGURE 3.5. Change in populations of villages over time.

3.5 presents the change in total populations. As part of the original study design, villages were matched on size, with two of the villages considerably larger than the other two.

Nuclear family size includes the mother and father and their offspring still living with them. Whereas in 1967 the mean nuclear family size per village ranged from 5.6 to 5.9, in 1974 the range was from 4.4 to 5.1. By 1987, the mean nuclear family size ranged from 4.6 to 5.0. In all the villages, mean nuclear family size decreased by about one person over the 20-year time span. In summary, there have been many improvements in the villages over the past 20 years, as evidenced by the positive changes in the measures just discussed. However, change has been slow, and given the starting point for most of the measures, these changes may not represent substantial reductions in the risks posed to child welfare. For example, between 1967 and 1987, the average number of years of schooling has approximately doubled in all the villages, but the increase in schooling is actually only about 1 year. Although positive, this increase will probably have only a minimal impact on children.

The Subjects

The sampling frame for this study is defined by the pool of subjects included in the longitudinal study ($N \approx 2,000$). All infant data used for the present analysis were selected based on the following criteria: full-term births (gestational age greater than or equal to 37

TABLE 3.1. Mean birthweight, birth length and length at 12 months of normal birthweight, symmetrical and asymetrical IUGR infants.

	Birth weight (g)	Length at birth (cm)	Length at 12 months (cm)
Normal birthweight	3,341	50.4	69.4
Symmetrical IUGR	2,768	48.2	67.9
Asymmetrical IUGR	2,650	50.5	69.2

TABLE 3.2. Proportion of sample from each village.

Village	IUGR	Normal birthweight
03	0.451	0.549
06	0.494	0.501
08	0.504	0.496
14	0.460	0.540

weeks), with available data on birth weight and body length at 15 days, available growth data at 12 months, and subsequent available data in 1988 ($N = 518$). Infants were classified as IUGR ($N = 248$) according to the standardized criteria proposed by the Centro Latinoamericano de Perinatologia (CLAP) (Schwarcz, Duverges, Diaz, & Fescina, 1986); that is, less than the 10th percentile for the weight distribution at a given gestational age. The remaining children with normal birthweight served as controls ($N = 270$).

IUGR subjects were then subdivided according to ponderal index (see definition below): low ponderal index (IUGR-LPI, $N = 80$) and adequate ponderal index (IUGR-API, $N = 168$).

Demographic and physical growth data for each of the three groups are presented in Tables 3.1 and 3.2. The proportion of the children that had IUGR is similar in all four villages. There is a striking difference in length at 12 months between the symmetrical IUGR infants and the other two groups. In addition, it should be noted that the mean age at which the children were tested in the cross-sectional study was similar in all three groups (NBW = 14.8 years, IUGR-API = 15.1 years, IUGR-LPI = 15.1 years).

CROSS-SECTIONAL DATA: 1988–1989

In June 1987, a follow-up study of the subjects included in the longitudinal study was undertaken. Over 80% were contacted and enrolled in the study. Data collection began in May 1988 and terminated in May 1989. The follow-up included data from the

Guatemalan Ministry of Education as well as classroom and school-level data containing complete schooling records for all children enrolled in school from 1976 to 1988 for the four experimental villages. Guatemalan children begin schooling at 7 years of age (at the earliest), hence children with infant data (born 1969 on) are matched with corresponding schooling data.

Variables and Measurements

INDEPENDENT VARIABLES

- Length of gestation: interval in weeks between the date of onset of the last menstrual period and the date of delivery.
- Birth weight: obtained within 24 hours after delivery.
- Body length: obtained at 15 days.
- Birth weight classification: IUGR defined as birth weight less than the 10th percentile for a given gestational age (CLAP, Schwarcz et al., 1986).
- Rohrer's Ponderal Index (PI): weight $\times$ 100/height^3 (Lubchenco, Hansman, & Boyd, 1966). This was calculated only for IUGR infants. A low PI (LPI) is characterized by below-average weight for average length. Where both measures are either high, average, or low, the PI is considered adequate. The cutoff point for LPI/API is the 10th percentile of the Lubchenco reference standards for 37 to 40 weeks gestation.
- Growth in the first 12 months: Since the purpose of entering growth in the model was to assess the contribution of growth in the first year of life independent of anthropometry at birth, a new variable was constructed in the following manner: The amount a subject grew in length during the first year was regressed on length at 15 days, and the residual, which represents the variance that could not be attributed to length at birth, was entered into the model as an independent variable.

DEPENDENT VARIABLES

A battery of psychoeducational tests was constructed to assess functional performance in adolescence. Specifically, the purpose was to evaluate intellectual capacities and abilities that may reflect both formal learning experiences as well as knowledge acquired in nonformal settings. The battery included reading, numeracy, general knowledge tests, and two educational achievement tests in reading and vocabulary. An overall measure of intelligence was obtained with Raven's Standard Progressive Matrices. The achievement tests were part of the Interamerican Series, which were constructed by the University of Texas, and have been used extensively in Guatemala and standardized by faculty from the Universidad del Valle in Guatemala City.

Tests of basic reading skills, numeracy, and general knowledge were administered individually by four trained testers. The achievement and intelligence tests were administered individually or in a group, depending on subject availability, time, and logistical constraints. The means and standard deviations for all of these variables broken down by birth weight classification are shown in Table 3.3.

All of the testers of functional performance were from Guatemala City or from another medium-sized city centrally located near the testing villages. They were females with certification as primary-level school teachers. All of the testers received extensive training by both Guatemalan and U.S. psychologists during pretesting and the pilot study.

Interrater reliability was calculated for reading, numeracy, and general knowledge tests based on four testing situations with five raters at each testing situation. Percent agreement varied between 86 and 100% for reading, 97 and 100% for numeracy, and 94 and 100% for general knowledge.

Specifics of the individual tests are described in detail below.

Literacy/Reading. The test consisted of two parts: (a) a preliteracy measure of knowledge of letters, syllables, words, and short phrases, and (b) a reading test based on material reflecting com-

TABLE 3.3. Mean numeracy, Raven's Progressive Matrices, reading, Interamerican reading and vocabulary scores by birth weight classification.

		Intrauterine growth retarded	
	Normal birthweight	Symmetrical	Asymmetrical
Numeracy	31.33 (8.92)	32.77 (7.43)	33.00 (7.93)
Raven's	10.43 (4.19)	10.39 (3.39)	11.76 (4.44)
Reading	14.94 (3.77)	15.23 (3.51)	15.51 (3.79)
Interamerican vocabulary	25.33 (7.18)	25.33 (7.15)	25.67 (8.55)
Interamerican reading	16.24 (4.49)	16.37 (4.73)	16.51 (5.18)

mon experiences of the subjects. Subjects with 4 years of schooling or less were given the prereading test, which was considered to be a screening test. The result of this test was a score on a scale of 1 to 4 (1 = unable to complete prereading test, suspended; 2 = completed test with at least five errors, suspended; 3 = completed test with less than five errors, continued; 4 = reading test administered directly).

The reading test consisted of 19 questions, which referred to two different sets of stimuli: a *cedula* (identification card) and related personal data, and a newspaper article on a soccer game. Coding of the literacy test was done by individual testers. Scoring was based on the total number of correct answers. The outcome variable, referred to as *reading* in this paper, reflects the reading test only and therefore includes only literate subjects.

Numeracy. The numeracy test measured ability to read numbers and prices, to sequence, and to solve problems. All subjects were asked to read aloud a list of numbers ranging from one to three digits, to read a list of prices of familiar articles, and to sequentially order a list of items with their prices. There were also three visual stimuli reflecting common situations of buying, working, and transportation. Subjects were asked to answer questions regarding costs, wages, fares, and distances that required the ability to add, subtract, multiply, or divide. There was a total of 41 items. Coding was done by individual testers, and scoring was based on the number of correct answers across all items.

General Knowledge. The knowledge test consisted of 22 questions regarding common experiences relating to schooling, work, transportation, legal-political structures, and health. Subjects were presented with situations requiring either basic knowledge or simple decision-making skills. Given three possible answers, they were asked to choose the response that they thought best answered the question. Coding was done by individual testers, and scoring reflected the total number of correct answers.

Achievement Tests. The Interamerican Reading Series is a standardized reading test originally designed to measure reading abilities of Spanish-speaking children in Texas. This test was chosen because of its previous use in Guatemala by researchers at the Universidad del Valle. The test consists of three parts: level of comprehension, speed of comprehension, and vocabulary. As a result of the pilot study, only the level of comprehension and vocabulary sections were included. All subjects who passed the preliteracy test, independent of years of schooling, were given the reading test. The tests were timed and given individually or in a group of up to four subjects. Subjects filled in circles on answer sheets. Scoring was the number of correct answers on each of the two scales: reading comprehension and vocabulary.

Intelligence. Intelligence level of all subjects was assessed by applying Raven's Standard Progressive Matrices. The test consists of five scales (A through E) of 12 items each. Each item contains a visual design with a piece missing. The subject is asked to select, from a possibility of six or eight patterns, the piece that completes the target design. Data from pilot testing suggested very low variance on sets D and E. Due to the level of difficulty and time constraints, sets A, B, and C were administered. Subjects worked at resolving the problems at their own rate. In the case of illiterate subjects the test was administered individually, and answers were coded by the testers.

Procedure

Each of the four villages was visited by a research team twice, once during the dry season and once during the rainy season. Research teams were rotated, and each team visited each village during one round of testing. The presence of the team in the village varied from 3 weeks to 9 weeks depending on the size of the village and coverage rates. Teams were made up of a doctor, two anthropometrists, several interviewers for sociodemographic data collection, and three persons trained to collect the behavioral data.

In each community, two individuals were hired to recruit subjects and make appointments for their attendance at the centers. All testing was done in community houses rented by the project and adapted for the specific testing situation. In addition to psychological data, subjects were given a medical examination and an anthropometric examination, and were interviewed regarding sociodemographic data.

Reliability

A primary goal of the assessment of reliability is to ensure that the variance associated with the testing instrument and the variance associated with the tester do not mask the interindividual variance related to the main effects proposed in the working hypothesis. Three types of reliability assessments (test-retest stability, internal homogeneity, and intertester differences) were carried out to determine the proportion of total score variance that was "error" variance, resulting from conditions irrelevant to the purpose of the test.

Test-Retest

Test-retest stability coefficients were assessed with a subsample of the Guatemalan adolescent study population ($N = 217$). The test-retest range was from 2 to 34 days with a mean range of 17.7 days (S.D. = 7.99). Tests that had a test-retest stability coefficient of less than .40 were dropped from further analyses.

Test-retest reliabilities were calculated using the Pearson Product Moment Coefficient. As can be seen in Table 3.4, the reliability coefficients for the functional competence tests are high, ranging from .85 to .90. Two of the functional competence tests, the Raven's Standard Progressive Matrices and the Interamerican Reading Series have published test-retest information from different populations and contexts. The Raven's, for example, is reported to have test-retest coefficients of .89, .81, and .78 (range 1 week, 1 month, and 3 months) for a subsample of Belgian school children (Stinissen, 1956), a coefficient of .82 (range of 7 to 10 days) for a population of Gold Coast teens (Jahoda, 1956), and a coefficient of .91 with Indian undergraduates (Rath, 1959). The coefficient in the Guatemalan population (.87) is similar to the published reliabilities. The retest reliability (alternate form) for the Interamerican Spanish version (reading and vocabulary combined)

TABLE 3.4. Test-retest correlations for functional competency tests.

Test	Pearson's correlation
Raven's ($N = 88$)	.87
Knowledge ($N = 87$)	.88
Interamerican ($N = 70$)	
Reading	.85
Vocabulary	.87
Reading Test ($N = 70$)	.88
Numeracy ($N = 89$)	.90

was .75 for a group of Spanish-speaking third graders in Puerto Rico (Manuel, 1967).

Internal Homogeneity

In addition to test-retest stability, error variance assessed internal homogeneity, demonstrating the consistency of a measure with regard to items and content.

Cronbach's alphas were calculated for internal consistency using the entire sample for the Raven's; the Interamerican series; and the knowledge, numeracy, and reading tests. The Raven's and the Interamerican vocabulary and reading tests had high Cronbach's alphas (.786 to .976), similar to internal consistency measures published in the literature for these tests. The Interamerican has a published internal consistency of .71 (total) based on a population of Spanish-speaking youths (Arnold, 1969). The consistency results for the Interamerican reading and vocabulary obtained in this study were much higher than those published (.98 and .95 respectively). The Raven's has published internal consistencies between .89 and .94 for school-age children in Belgium and Iran (Baraheni, 1974; Stinissen, 1956; Swinnen, 1958).

The internal homogeneity for the numeracy, knowledge, and reading tests were of particular interest, as these tests were constructed specifically for use with the Guatemalan adolescents. The alpha for the numbers test was .95, suggesting high internal consistency. Alpha coefficients for the knowledge test (.67) and the reading test (.75) were not as robust but were still within the acceptable range for internal consistency. Item deletion in some cases increased the coefficient only marginally and hence was not considered necessary for subsequent analyses.

Data Analysis

The general linear model with a Type III sum of squares in an analysis of covariance format was used to estimate mean and interactive effects (SAS, 5th ed., 1985). This type of analysis was used because the hypotheses to be tested are invariant to the order of the effects, and the hypothesis for one effect does not involve the hypothesis for another effect. The number of cases varies between analyses; accordingly, the respective means differ, as determined by the number of subjects included in each analysis.

Results

Table 3.5 presents the F-values for the models and the independent variables for the five dependent variables described above. This first set of results represents the comparison of those subjects with IUGR and normal birthweight for gestational age. All of the models explained a significant proportion of the variance in the outcome variables. Consistently, the five analyses yielded statistically significant main effects of growth and no effects of birthweight. The slopes in the regression shown in Table 3.6 indicate that the more a child grew in length in the first year of life (independent of length at birth), the higher his or her scores on the Raven's Standard Progressive Matrices, the Interamerican reading and vocabulary tests, and the numeracy and reading tests. On the other hand, test performance did not differ between the subjects with IUGR and those with normal birth weight. The interaction of birth weight classification and growth in the first year of life was significant only in the case of the numeracy test (see Figure 3.6). It can be seen from the regression line that growth is not associated with the numeracy scores in the normal birth weight group. In contrast, within the IUGR group, the more a child grew in the first year of life, the higher his numeracy test score.

TABLE 3.5. Summary table of results (F-values) of general linear model regressions.[1]

	Raven's	Reading	Interamerican Vocabulary	Interamerican Reading	Numeracy
Model	6.01*	3.52***	7.83*	5.79**	3.64***
Birth weight classification	0.48	0.59	0.19	0.07	2.68
Growth	17.54*	10.38**	22.08*	16.74*	3.56****
Birth weight class * Growth	0.97	0.44	1.21	0.09	6.52***

* $p < .001$
** $p < .01$
*** $p < .05$
**** $.05 > p < .10$
[1] For Raven Progressive Matrices, Interamerican reading and vocabulary achievement tests, numeracy, and reading test scores by birth weight classification (normal birth weight versus IUGR infants).
Sample sizes are as follows: NBW = 177; IUGR = 169 (may vary slightly depending on outcome).

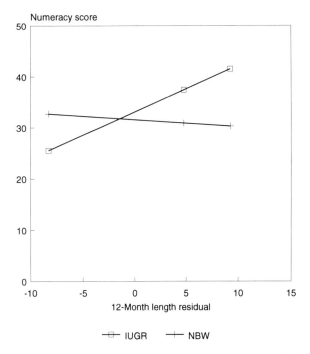

FIGURE 3.6. Regression of numeracy on growth for IUGR and NBW infants (NBW = normal birthweight).

Another set of analyses was performed to identify possible statistical differences between symmetrical and asymmetrical cases within the IUGR group. Table 3.7 presents the *F*-values for the models and the independent variables for the outcome variables described above. The primary issue is not the differences between these two subgroups but possible interactions between body proportions and growth at 12 months that could have remained undetected by the series of previous analyses. For the Raven's Standard Progressive Matrices the main effects of ponderal index and growth were statistically significant (Table 3.7). This main effect of body proportions on the Raven's Standard Progressive Matrices scores indicates that subjects with asymmetrical IUGR performed significantly better than those with symmetrical IUGR (*p* < .01). In contrast, there were no main effects of body proportions on either reading or vocabulary achievement scores or on the

TABLE 3.6. Slopes showing the effect of length velocity in the first year of life on dependent variables.

Dependent variable	Slope in regression
Raven's	0.51*
Interamerican reading (achievement test)	0.61*
Interamerican vocabulary (achievement test)	0.93*
Numeracy test	0.91*
Reading test	0.43**

*$p < .01$
**$p < .05$

TABLE 3.7. Summary table of results (F-values) of general linear model regressions.[1]

	Raven's	Achievement tests		Reading	Numeracy
		Reading	Vocabulary		
Model	7.41*	2.59***	2.85**	2.43	3.94*
Ponderal index (PI)	7.54*	0.39	0.17	0.44	0.07
Growth	15.82*	7.49*	8.07*	7.01*	11.67*
PI *growth	2.38	0.74	1.61	0.34	1.89

*$p < .01$
**$p < .05$
***$.05 < p < .10$
[1] For Raven's Progressive Matrices, Interamerican reading and vocabulary achievement tests, numeracy, and reading test scores for symmetrical and asymmetrical IUGR infants.

numeracy and reading tests. However, there were main effects of growth during the first 12 months of life on these variables. Table 3.8 shows that the more linear growth exhibited in the first year (controlling for birth length), the higher the scores on the Raven's Standard Progressive Matrices, the Interamerican achievement tests, and the numeracy test.

Discussion

The IUGR subjects of the present study were born into a nutritionally at-risk population, with low levels of formal education and

TABLE 3.8. Slopes showing the effect of length velocity in the first year of life on dependent variables in the model.[1]

Dependent variable	Slope in regression
Raven's	0.82*
Interamerican reading (achievement test)	0.86***
Interamerican vocabulary (achievement test)	1.49**
Numeracy test	1.44**
Reading test	0.56***

*$p < .001$
**$p < .01$
***$p < .05$
[1] Includes only symmetrical and asymmetrical subjects.

an economically impoverished rural environment. On this same group of subjects Martorell, Yarbrough, Lechtig, Habicht, and Klein (1975) (see also Yarbrough, Habicht, Malina, Lechtig, & Klein, 1975) observed severe growth retardation during weaning and a high incidence of infection, particularly diarrhea. Social and economic improvements have occurred in the four villages over the last 20 years, but the quality of housing is still unsatisfactory, as judged by housing structure and types of floor, water systems, and methods of human waste disposal. Similarly, while the number of illiterate women has decreased significantly, 30% or more of the women remain illiterate in each village.

Within such a population and environmental context it was expected that IUGR would leave developmental sequelae that would be clearly detectable in adolescence. In fact, we had proposed that under those circumstances IUGR was likely to be an important determinant of the child's developmental trajectory because of adverse environmental conditions. It was further hypothesized that among IUGR cases the highest risk would be found among those subjects who were also growth retarded after birth. However, we found no support for either assertion. Likewise, we found no evidence that body symmetry at birth increased the developmental risk of IUGR. Regardless of whether the causality of IUGR was a poor supply of nutrients to the fetus throughout pregnancy or a particular nutritional insult in the last trimester of pregnancy, it was clear that IUGR did not represent a developmental risk in terms of adolescent functional performance. At issue is what factors safeguarded the development of the IUGR subjects.

The social and family environment of the subjects is not likely to have played a major preventative or remedial role. Support for this assumption is found in the description of poor environmental conditions and, more important, in the fact that in most cases the continuity of pre- and postnatal growth retardation did not increase the developmental risk of the IUGR cases. There is ample evidence that postnatal growth retardation is a sign not only of poor nutrition and poor health but also of an environment that fails to meet children's social, emotional, and educational needs (Pollitt & Ricciuti, 1969; Ricciuti, 1981b; Ricciuti, 1989; Grantham-McGregor, 1984; Mosley & Chen, 1984). Accordingly, in the present circumstances, it can be assumed that in at least a few IUGR cases with postnatal growth retardation the environment was less than optimal. Yet we did not find that the pre- and postnatal growth retarded subjects were at any greater disadvantage than those who were retarded only in growth after birth.

Age has been considered a powerful developmental factor, since the probabilities of finding developmental deficits associated to early trauma decrease significantly as the child grows older (Sameroff & Chandler, 1975). In another paper we reported cognitive development data at 36, 48, and 60 months of the symmetrical IUGR infants included in the present analysis (Gorman & Pollitt, in press). In that study, postnatal growth retardation data were also included in the analysis. At 36 months, IUGR did show an independent association in the expected direction with verbal cognitive abilities. At 36 and 48 months there was also an interaction between IUGR and postnatal growth in the performance on measures of short-term memory. As growth retardation increased, the probabilities of finding comparatively poor memory scores in the IUGR subjects also increased. However, by 60 months no adverse effects of IUGR were detected on either verbal ability or memory.

Conjointly, the data from the assessments at 36, 48, and 60 months and the data from the present analysis suggest that as the child grows older the probabilities of detecting developmental deviations seem to decrease. Whereas IUGR subjects were at a disadvantage in all areas tested at 36 months, they showed no specific deficits in adolescence.

In contrast to our original expectation that postnatal growth retardation would increase the developmental risk of IUGR, we found that IUGR subjects who grew more rapidly in the first year of life tended to perform better than all other subjects on a numeracy test. We have no readily available explanation for this surprising finding. Speculatively, it could be argued that in order for the IUGR cases to have grown well during the first year of life they must have been exposed to a favorable social and family environment that could have also been beneficial to their cognitive development. However, this argument is weakened by the absence of a similar test performance pattern among the subjects with normal birth weight who grew well in the first year of life.

The role of body proportions at birth among the IUGR children was also unexpected. There was no evidence that either symmetrical or asymmetrical IUGR subjects were at a greater disadvantage as compared to the normal birth weight subjects. In fact, in contrast to our predictions, a comparison of the Raven's test scores of symmetrical IUGR, asymmetrical IUGR, and normal birth weight infants suggested that whereas there was no difference between the symmetrical IUGR and the normal birth weight infants, the asymmetrical IUGR subjects were better-off as compared to the normal birth weight subjects. Here again, we have no explanation for this particular finding, except to suggest that it may be due to chance.

Before turning to a discussion of the effects of postnatal growth, it is important to recognize that this study did not explore the role of severity of IUGR. It seems biologically plausible that a more stringent definition of IUGR (e.g., based on the 5th percentile for a given weight distribution at a given gestational age) would have yielded different outcomes from those observed. A recent report of the National Academy of Sciences (1990) on nutrition in pregnancy underscores this issue and points to the need to discriminate between developmental outcomes of IUGR as a function of severity. However, it is also important to recognize that the definition of IUGR used in the present study is standard.

Although there was no evidence that IUGR was associated with a developmental deviation, there was strong evidence that growth retardation during the first year of life covaried with poor performance in all of the tests administered. This is to a large extent an expected finding. Although there are probably very few studies in the world that have reported associations between size in infancy and functional performance in adolescence, it is well established that growth retardation in childhood covaries with low IQ, poor cognitive test performance, and low school achievement (Pollitt, 1990). As we have suggested earlier, however, these findings cannot be attributed to any one particular nutritional, health, or social environmental set of factors. Growth faltering in early life has been associated with protein energy malnutrition, iron deficiency, high incidence of morbidity, and numerous other social factors such as poor maternal education and extreme poverty (Mosley & Chen, 1984). All of these factors may well have contributed in different degrees to the deficits observed.

As may have been already inferred, we assume that the differences observed in the effects of pre- and postnatal growth retardation are not due to a differential risk associated with particular developmental periods or the nature of a particular causal factor. We interpret these differences to mean that, whereas IUGR is likely to be secondary to nutritional factors (National Academy of Sciences, 1990), postnatal growth retardation is not likely to depend solely on nutritional factors but on other health and social factors as well. In Guatemala, for example, Mata (1978) has shown that during the first year of life the frequency and severity of gastrointestinal, respiratory, and other infections are closely related to weight gain. In the United States, nonorganic failure to thrive has been associated with multiple causal factors at different levels of the ecological context of the child, involving socioenvironmental conditions such as problems in mother-child interaction and disturbances in feeding (Pollitt, 1988).

It follows that prenatal nutritional stress may not be sufficient to produce long-term developmental deviations. On the other hand, the multiple factors involved in the causation of growth retardation in early postnatal life do compromise other developmental domains such as cognition and school aptitudes.

In summary, there does not seem to be an empirical basis from which to postulate that the long-term developmental outcomes of IUGR children will differ in developing as compared to developed countries. In both instances, the developmental deviations that may be observed in infancy and the early childhood period seem to disappear over time, and few, if any, functional differences seem to exist between subjects with and without IUGR by the time of their adolesence.

Acknowledgments. Supported in part by grants from the March of Dimes (grant #12–238) and the National Institutes of Child Health and Human Development (grant #HD22440). We gratefully acknowledge the contribution of the Institute of Nutrition of Central America and Panama (INCAP) for their important role in the data collection for this project. The study was a collaborative effort involving several institutions: R. Martorell (Principal Investigator; originally at Stanford, now at Cornell University), J. Rivera (INCAP, Guatemala), E. Pollitt (U.C.Davis), and Jere Haas (Cornell University).

References

Adair, L., & Pollitt, E. (1985). Outcome of maternal nutritional supplementation: A comprehensive review of the Bacon Chow study. *American Journal of Clinical Nutrition, 41*, 948–978.

Arnold, D. (1969). Reliability of test scores for the young "bilingual" disadvantaged. *Reading Teacher, 22*(4), 341–345.

Baraheni, M.N. (1974). Raven's Progressive Matrices as applied to Iranian children. *Educational and Psychological Measurement, 34*, 983–988.

Belizán, J.M., & Villar, J. (1988). El crecimiento fetal y su repercusión sobre el desarrollo del niño. In M. Cusminsky, E.M. Moreno, y E.N. Suarez Ojeda, (Eds.), *Crecimiento y Desarrollo: Hechos y tendencias.* Pan American Health Organization. Scientific Publication No. 510:102–119.

Friedman, S.L., & Sigman, M. (Eds.). (1981). *Preterm birth and psychological development.* New York: Academic Press.

Grantham-McGregor, S. (1984). Social background of childhood malnutrition. In J. Brozek, & B. Schurch (Eds.), *Malnutrition and behavior: critical assessment of key issues.* Lausanne, Switzerland: Nestlé Foundation.

Gorman, K., & Pollitt, E. (in press). The relationship between weight and body proportionality at birth, growth during the first year of life, and cognitive development at 36, 48 and 60 months. *Infant Behavior and Development.*

Haas, J.D., Balcazar, H., & Caulfield, L. (1987). Variation in early neonatal mortality for different types of fetal growth retardation. *American Journal of Physical Anthropology, 73*, 467–473.

Hack, M., & Breslau, N. (1988). Biologic and social determinants of 3-year IQ in very low birthweight children. In P. Vietze & H.G. Vaughan (Eds.) *Early identification of infants with developmental disabilities.* Orlando, FL: Grune & Stratton.

Halas, E.S. (1983). Behavioral changes accompanying zinc deficiency in animals. In I.E. Dreosti & R.M. Smith, (Eds.), *Neurobiology of the trace elements, Vol. 1: Trace element neurobiology and deficiencies* (pp. 213–243).

Clifton, NJ: Humana Press.

Hill, R.M., Veniaud, W.M., Deter, R.L., Tennyson, L.M., Rettig, G.M., Zion, T.E., Vorderman, A.L., Helms, P.G., McCulley, L.B., & Hill L.L. (1984). The effect of intrauterine malnutrition on the term infant: A 14-year progressive study. *Acta Paediatrica Scandinavica, 73*, 482–487.

Jahoda, G. (1956). Assessment of abstract behavior in a non-Western culture. *Journal of Abnormal Social Psychology, 53*, 237–243.

Joos, S., & Pollitt, E. (1984). Effects of supplementation on behavioral development in children up to the age of two years: A comparison of four studies. In J., Brozek & B. Schurch (Eds.), *Malnutrition and behavior: Critical assessment of key issues* (pp. 507–519). Lausanne, Switzerland: The Nestlé Foundation.

Lin, C.C., & Evans, M.I. (1984). *Intrauterine growth retardation: Pathophysiology and clinical management.* New York: McGraw-Hill.

Lohman, T.G., Roche, A.F., & Martorell, R. (Eds.). (1988). *Anthropometric standardization reference manual.* Human Kinetics Publishers.

Lozoff, B. (1989). Iron deficiency and infant behavior *American Journal of Clinical Nutrition, 50*(3), suppl., 641–651.

Lubchenco, L., Hansman, C., & Boyd, E. (1966). Intrauterine growth in length and head circumference as estimated from live birth at gestational ages from 26 to 42 weeks. *Pediatrics, 37*, 403–408.

Manuel, H. (1967). *Technical report, tests of general ability and tests of reading: Interamerican series.* San Antonio, TX: Guidance Testing Associates.

Martorell, R., Delgado, H.J., Valverde, V., & Klein, R.E. (1981). Maternal stature, fertility and infant mortality. *Human Biology, 53*, 303–312.

Martorell, R., & Habicht, J-P. (1986). Growth in early childhood in developing countries. In F. Faltner & J.M. Tanner (Eds.), *Human growth: A comprehensive treatise, Vol. 3*: Methodology: ecological, genetic, and nutritional effects on growth (2nd ed., pp. 241–262). New York: Plenum Press.

Martorell, R., Yarbrough C., Lechtig, A., Habicht, J.P., & Klein R.E. (1975). Diarrheal disease and growth retardation in preschool Guatemalan children. *American Journal of Physical Anthropology, 43*, 341–346.

Mata, L. (1978). *The children of Santa Maria Cauque.* Cambridge, MA: MIT Press.

Mosley, H., & Chen, L. (Eds.). (1984). *Child survival: Strategies for research.* London: Cambridge University Press.

Mueller, W.H., & Pollitt, E. (1984). The Bacon Chow Study: Effects of maternal nutrition supplementation on birth measurements of children, accounting for the size of a previous (unsupplemented) child. *Early Human Development, 10*, 127–136.

National Academy of Sciences. (1990). *Nutrition during pregnancy.* Washington, DC: National Academy Press.

Ounsted, M.K., Moar, V.A., & Scott R. (1986). Growth and proportionality in early childhood, Vol. 3: Differences between babies of low birth weight in well-nourished and malnourished populations. *Early Human Development*, 1, 167–178.

Pilch, S.M., & Senti, F.R. (1984). Assessment of iron nutritional status of the U.S. population based on data collected in the second national health and nutrition examination survey, 1976–1980.

Pollitt, E. (1983). Morbidity and infant development: A hypothesis. *International Journal of Behavioral Development*, 6, 461–475.

Pollitt, E. (1988). Developmental impact of nutrition in pregnancy, infancy and childhood: Public health issues in the United States. In N.W. Bray (Ed.), *International Review of Mental Retardation*, 15 (pp. 33–80). New York: Academic press.

Pollitt, E. (1990). *Malnutrition and infection in the classroom*. Paris: United Nations Educational, Scientific and Cultural Organization.

Pollitt, E., & Riccuiti, H. (1969). Biological and social correlates of stature among children in the slums of Lima, Peru. *Americal Journal of Orthopsychiatry*, 39(5), 735–747.

Rantakallio, P. (1985). A 14-year follow-up of children with normal and abnormal birth weight for their gestational age. *Acta Paediatrica Scandinavica*, 74, 62–69.

Rath, R. (1959). Standardisation of Progressive Matrices among college students. *Journal of Vocational and Educational Guidance*, 5(4), 167–171.

Ricciuti, H.N. (1981b). Developmental consequences of malnutrition in early childhood. In M. Lewis & L.A. Rosenblum (Eds.), *The uncommon child: The genesis of behavior* (Vol. 3, pp. 151–172). New York: Plenum Press.

Ricciuti, H.N. (1989). Malnutrition and cognitive development: Research-policy linkages and current research directions. In R.J. Sternberg & L. Okagaki (Eds.), *Directors of development: Influences on the development of children's thinking*.

Sameroff, A.J., & Chandler, M.J. (1975). Reproductive risk and the continuum of caretaking casualty. In F.D. Horowitz, (Ed.), *Review of child development research* (pp. 187–244). Chicago: The University of Chicago Press.

SAS Institute, Inc. (1989). *SAS users guide: Statistics version 6*, 4th ed. Cary, NC: SAS Institute.

Schwarcz, R., Duverges, C., Diaz, A.G., & Fescina, R.H. (1986). *Obstetricia*, 4th ed. Buenos Aires: El Ateneo.

Stinissen, J. (1956). De warrde van de Progressive Matrices 38: Een vieuwe vorm voor de lagere school [The value of Progressive Matrices 38: A new form for elementary school.] *Tijdscher stud-Beropsurient*, 3, 102–124.

Swinnen, K. (1958). Een onderzoekment de Progressive Matrices '38 op een goep leerlingen van de zesde latijuse en zesde moderne. *Tijdschrift voor Studie und Beroepsorienterung*, 5, 13–25.

Thomson, C.A., & Pollitt E. (1977). Effects of severe protein-calorie malnutrition on behavior in human populations. In L. Greene (Ed.), *Malnutrition, behavior and social organization*. New York: Academic Press.

Townsend, J., Klein, R.E., Irwin, C., Owens, W., Yarbrough, C., & Engle, P. (1982). Nutrition and preschool mental development. In D.A. Wagner & H.W. Stevenson (Eds.), *Cultural perspective on child development*. San Francisco: Freeman.

Vietze, P.M., & Vaughan, H.G. (1988). *Early identification of infants with developmental disabilities*. Philadelphia: Grunne Straton.

Villar, J., & Belizan, J.M. (1982). The relative contribution of prematurity and fetal growth retardation to low birth weight in developing and developed societies. *American Journal of Obstetrics and Gynecology, 143,* 793–798.

Villar, J., Smeriglio, V., Martorell, R., Brown, C.H., & Klein, R.E. (1984). Heterogeneous growth and mental development of intrauterine growth-retarded infants during the first three years of life. *Pediatrics, 74*(5), 783–791.

Werner, E.E., & Smith, R.S. (1977). *Kauai's children come of age*. Honolulu: University Press of Hawaii.

Westwood, M., Kramer, M., Munz, D., Lovett, J.M., & Watters, G.M. (1983). Growth and development of full-term nonasphyxiated small-for-gestational-age newborns: Follow-up through adolescence. *Pediatrics, 71,* 376–382.

Winick M., & Meyer R.C. (1975). Malnutrition and environmental enrichment by early adoption. *Science, 190,* 1173–1175.

Yarbrough, C., Habicht, J.P., Malina, R.M., Lechtig, A., & Klein, R.E. (1975). Length and weight in rural Guatemalan Ladino children, birth to 7 years of age. *American Journal of Physical Anthropology, 42,* 439–448.

4
Infant Predictors of Inhibited and Uninhibited Children

Jerome Kagan and Nancy Snidman

Introduction

Explanations of the variation in human behavior, especially those qualities that a culture regards as prototypic of the ideal, are high on the list of preoccupations of the citizen as well as those whose role it is to provide scientifically valid interpretations. The philosophical premises of each culture direct, often in subtle ways, the preferred interpretations, whereas available evidence, no matter how primitive, constrains theorists from generating potentially valid explanations that few will accept because the mind needs scaffolding for arguments that rest on novel or unpopular premises.

Democracies, whether of classical Athens or contemporary Washington, D.C., usually prefer interpretations of behavior that maximize the power of the environment, because such arguments imply malleability in human character and therefore sustain the hope for a progressive increase in human happiness and dignity. The Greeks supposed that variation in diet and climate were potent; Americans are equally certain that experiences in the family during the early years of life are influential. The scientific evidence, if we can call the data available to Hippocrates scientific, made a belief in climate and diet reasonable to the Greeks, whereas the facts of modern behaviorism made environmental explanations palatable to us.

A society that is more hierarchical is more likely to accept relatively permanent divisions among the members of its population and to be receptive to explanations that award power to endogenous qualities of the person. It is not a coincidence that the 18th- and 19th-century constitutional explanations of behavior had a greater appeal on the continent than in England, because class and ethnic divisions seemed to continental Europeans to rest on fixed rather than conventional qualities.

As I have written elsewhere, if it were not for the egalitarianism of the many Americans who wanted to believe that the new arrivals from Europe were, despite their language, dress, and habits, no different from themselves, we might not have rejected these constitutional ideas and taken up behaviorism with such avidity. I fear that the growing acceptance of the role of biological processes on personality, which I am going to discuss today, reflects an easy willingness to accept the fact that women can never be exactly like men and dark-skinned citizens never like Caucasians. I believe, as you shall see, that a child's biological qualities make a significant contribution to his or her character and behavior, but the dynamics of a life are so complex and the typical demands on each person in our society so well within his or her capacity that the fact of biological influence has no ethical or legal implications. To put it plainly, in the context of the women's movement, even though it is likely that science will discover that mammalian females are slightly more prone to states of anxiety than males, it does not follow that any vocation or role in modern society should be closed to them. After all, tall men perform significantly better in basketball than short ones, yet no one is suggesting that men under 5'10" be barred from the sport, because we all recognize that persistent effort and will often overcome biology.

The Idea of Temperament

It is common for humans to invent special words to name aspects of human nature while marking similar phenomena in animals with a different term. Such a linguistic strategy maintains a distinctiveness between us and them. Strains of animals within a species differ in body form, behavior, and physiology. Scott and Fuller (1965) showed that fearful behavior varied among species of dogs; Mason and his colleagues (Clarke, Mason, & Moberg, 1988) have demonstrated a similar result in rhesus, pigtail, and crabeater macaque monkeys. The closest concept to that of strain in humans is the idea of race. But the strong egalitarian ethic in America, and the fact that the reproductive isolation of the first 50,000 years of Homo sapiens is over, have led biologists to conclude, correctly, that the idea of race is not theoretically useful, even though these same biologists acknowledge that certain African populations are prone to develop sickle-cell anemia and that Asians have difficulty metabolizing alcohol.

The word *temperament*, which has a long history, has returned, although some of its older features have taken on a special meaning over the last 200 years. Originally, the word *temperament* was meant to refer to the fundamental, minimally plastic qualities of a person, while not implying that their origin was heredity. Today, the term *temperament* is similar in meaning to the word *strain* in animals. Temperament refers to a coherent profile of correlated physiological, physical, and behavioral qualities that are derived from a discrete genotype. Infants are born with different physiological and behavioral profiles, and their environments act on these profiles to produce, over time, a temperamental type. The profiles present on the first day of life are not temperamental types; they are the anlage of these types. The word *temperament* refers to the coherent product that emerges as a child's biologically based characteristics encounter experience. Thus, no baby is born an introverted temperamental type. This use of words is similar to use of the word *schizophrenia*. A child born to two schizophrenic parents, who therefore is likely to become schizophrenic in late adolescence, is not schizophrenic at birth, even though that child may possess the genes that place her at high risk for that category. The term *schizophrenia* is applied only after a profile of symptoms emerges as a result of experiences. The same logic implies to diseases with known genetic predispositions, like diabetes, cancer, and Huntington's chorea. A symptom-free 10-year-old who will develop Huntington's chorea at age 40 because he has the gene is not yet placed in that fateful category.

It is not clear how many temperamental types there will be. I suspect that the number is potentially very large, for a majority of genes contribute to the structure and physiology of the central nervous system. One likely set of mechanisms that influence behavior and mood are the hormones, peptides, and neurotransmitters produced by the brain. The number of such chemicals is estimated to be between 100 and 200, and the estimate is likely to become larger. It is also probable that the concentrations of most of these chemicals are controlled by a small number of genes. Thus, the chemical composition of the broth in which the brain sits is genetically influenced, and the number of functionally distinct broths is very large. Further, most of these broths determine the firing pattern of specific parts of the brain. As an example, the level of central norepinephrine affects, in a serious way, the excitability of sites in the limbic system, which, in turn, influences mood and behavior. I believe these chemical broths are the most important bases of a temperamental type. In an argument analogous to the one used by immunologists to categorize four types of allergies, I suggest that Type 1 temperamental categories refer to stable psychological profiles that have their origin in the chemical broths in which the brain sits. This statement is analogous to saying that Type 1 allergies are those in which there are high levels of immunoglobulin E.

The number of temperamental types will be much larger than the number that is discussed today, and these categories will refer to diverse aspects of human function—affective, behavioral, and intellectual. Unusual artistic ability, for example, may be as much a temperamental quality as a dour, melancholic demeanor. Because physiologists have yet to discover the basic neurochemical profiles that are the origins of temperamental categories, it will be necessary for psychologists to be inductive in their work and to infer these categories from rich corpora of behavioral and biological evidence. In light of the available information, I do not believe one can decide on an exhaustive set of categories a priori, although this is a popular strategy. Some psychologists have suggested that there is a small number of basic temperamental categories— sociability, neuroticism, anxiety, and activity level are usually high on most lists. This premature closure is similar to the Greek attempt at simplification by deciding that air, water, fire, and earth were the four basic natural elements. It is easy to understand why contemporary scholars are motivated to reduce all of the variation to a few constructs. The phenomena of interest are so complicated that it is reassuring to assume that three to six categories will account for all of the variance.

There is, in addition, a methodological problem in this work that is independent of the issue of the number of temperamental types. This problem involves the source of evidence. Over 90 percent of the studies of human temperament use interviews and questionnaires as the only source of information. The problem with this strategy is that this method relies on words that are understandable to the subjects in the study. Because it is unlikely that the final set of valid categories will be described easily with our current vocabulary, this method must be supplemented now, and eventually replaced. Suppose 18th- and 19th-century taxonomists relied on the verbal reports of people who knew a great deal about animals—trappers, breeders, farmers—as their main source of evidence for classification. These informants would never have placed dolphins and foxes in a similar class nor decided that bees, spiders, and lobsters were phylogenetic kin. I believe that, at the moment, we must be Baconian, as Linnaeus and his immediate successors were, and infer the basic temperamental types from behavioral and biological evidence. If one adopts this atheoretical posture, which always holds the danger of becoming empirically barbaric, it is likely that the first discoveries will be the most obvious and the easiest to quantify. This fact does not mean that the initial categories are the best exemplars of temperament, the most stable, or even the ones that are inherited in a simple way. It only means that they are obvious to observers—as the periodicity of the moon was to the Egyptians and the Mayans.

Inhibited and Uninhibited Children

The initial behavior of children and adults in unfamiliar situations, especially with unfamiliar people, is one such obvious phenomenon that is of interest to parents, teachers, and employers. That is why Jung (1924) claimed that the extravert and introvert were basic types, why Eysenck (1953) postulated extroversion/introversion as one of his two basic personality dimensions, and why Schneirla (1965) argued that approach and withdrawal were the basic differentiating dimensions among animals.

My colleagues and I have been studying two types of children who exemplify these two different styles when they encounter unfamiliar events. We do not regard these two types as falling on a continuum, even though it is easy to place scores indexing approach-avoidance on a continuum. But it is also easy to place adult reports of sadness or children's IQ scores on a phenotypic continuum, even though we know that the bipolar depressive is a distinct category of person qualitatively different from one who temporarily reports a blue mood, and a Down's syndrome child with an IQ of 75 is qualitatively different from an economically disadvantaged child with a normal complement of chromosomes whose IQ is 76.

We believe that inhibited and uninhibited children, our names for the two types, are qualitatively different because the physiological mechanisms that predispose a child to become inhibited at 2 years of age are not the complement of those mechanisms that predispose a child to become uninhibited. However, we recognize that this suggestion is not supported by sufficient evidence at the present time.

A series of previously published papers contain three robust facts. First, about 15% of Caucasian 2-year-old children living in relatively secure working-class or middle-class homes are consistently and extremely shy, timid, and emotionally restrained when they encounter unfamiliar events and people, and about 25% show the opposite profile. Second, these two groups maintain their respective temperamental styles, to a significant degree, through late childhood. We have followed these children through 7.5 years and found that about half of the inhibited children retain a timid, shy, demeanor and that over three quarters of the uninhibited children preserve their spontaneity and sociability. In our earlier work with the Fels longitudinal population, these qualities were preserved to a significant degree through adulthood.

Third, the two temperamental groups differ on peripheral physiological measures that imply differential reactivity in limbic sites, especially the amygdala and hypothalamus. The inhibited children show signs of greater sympathetic reactivity, as evidenced by larger pupillary dilations, less variable heart rates, and larger heart-rate accelerations to mild cognitive stress. Recently we have been examining the variation in vasoconstriction of the capillaries of the face in inhibited and uninhibited children. These children, who are now 10 to 11 years old, were originally selected to be inhibited or uninhibited when they were 21 or 31 months. We recorded the profiles of temperatures on the face using an Agema thermography scanner while the child sat in an internal room of a building whose temperature ranged from 70 to 73 degrees Fahrenheit. The protocol began with a recording of two baseline images followed by eight images in which the child listened to strings of six digits recorded on tape, knowing that he or she was to repeat these strings of digits after each series had been completed. We chose a digit recall task because of prior research indicating that such a task is perceived as stressful and because Nancy Braverman, in her Radcliffe senior honors thesis (1989), had found different patterns of vasoconstriction in introverted and extroverted female college students who were given a similar task.

During the analytic phase, the coder first retrieved each facial image on the computer screen. She then placed a rectangular form on the forehead so that the form avoided the hairline and was to the left and right of the midline of the face. A second pair of rectangles was placed about 1 centimeter below the first pair and covered the area of the eyes.

The temperature of the skin is influenced by the amount of blood in the capillaries that serve the epidermis. The amount of blood in these capillaries is under the partial control of arteriovenous anastomoses, which have muscular coats innervated by vaso-constrictor nerve fibers, which secrete norepinephrine and involve alpha noradrenergic receptors. When these sympathetic fibers serving the anastomoses are innervated, the muscles constrict; less blood flows to the capillaries; and, as a result, the skin becomes cooler. These anastomoses are most dense on the feet, hands, and lips, and in the area around the eyes and nose.

Recent research suggests that sympathetic innervation of the cardiovascular system is greater on the right than on the left side, implying that subjects with greater sympathetic tone should show greater cooling on the right than on the left side. This predicted asymmetry is in accord with the recent work of Richard Davidson and his colleagues (Davidson & Fox, 1989; Davidson & Tomarken, 1989), who have shown that fearful infants and children have greater suppression of alpha in the EEG on the right frontal pole than on the left (i.e., greater activation on the right than on the left side). These preliminary results affirm the greater sympathetic tone of inhibited children and imply that inhibited children have greater activation in limbic sites on the right side of the brain.

We have seen 66 children who had been inhibited or uninhibited at 21 or 31 months of age.

More inhibited children showed greater cooling on the right than on the left side of the face to the cognitive stress of digit recall. When an inhibited child showed cooling to digit recall, he or she was more likely to cool on the right side of the face, compared to baseline values, whereas more uninhibited children showed their greatest cooling on the left side.

The inhibited children also show signs of greater muscle tension, as evidenced by postural tone and reduced variability of the pitch periods of vocal utterances. The latter reflects greater muscle tension in the larynges and vocal cords. Finally, the inhibited children show consistently higher levels of salivary cortisol over the period of 5.5 to 7.5 years of age. Although the uninhibited children showed the opposite qualities, the association between temperamental type and physiology is always better for the uninhibited children. That is, low and variable heart rates, low levels of muscle tension, and low cortisol levels are more characteristic of uninhibited children than high levels are for inhibited ones.

We have interpreted these facts as indicating that the threshold of excitability of the amygdala and its projections to the hypothalamus, corpus striatum, and autonomic nervous system are more excitable and that the basis of this differential excitability is neurochemical. The most relevant chemical candidates are norepinephrine, corticotropin-releasing hormone endogenous opioids, or the density of receptors for these chemicals on neurons in the amygdala and the hypothalamus. These speculative suggestions are, of course, not yet affirmed.

Infant Predictors

A reasonable reply to these conclusions, especially if one is committed to an environmental view of personality, is that the children who differed in their degree of fearfulness at 2 years of age were socialized to behave this way and, as a consequence of their differential socialization, displayed the peripheral physiological qualities we found. In order to answer this reasonable criticism, it is necessary to study the young infant. We are now engaged in such a project, and the remainder of this paper summarizes our preliminary results.

The rationale for the procedures we implemented came from a serendipitous discovery by Lipsitt and his colleagues (LaGasse, Gruber, & Lipsitt, 1989) at Brown University. They found that the newborns who showed a dramatic increase in sucking rate when the water they were sucking suddenly turned sweet (by adding sucrose) were more likely to be inhibited in the second year than those newborns who did not show a major increase in sucking rate when the taste quality of the water changed suddenly. Physiologists tell us that the change in sweetness, as well as changes in all sensory modalities, are processed first by the cortex and then the amygdala. Information from every sensory modality eventually arrives at the amygdala. Further, the amygdala can be the origin of changes in motor activity—like sucking—as well as changes in the sympathetic nervous system and the hypothalamic-pituitary-adrenal axis. Thus, we presented to a large number of infants changes in visual, auditory, and olfactory events to see which of them showed large and which small changes in behavior, with the hope that the variation in behavioral arousal would reveal which infants were born with an excitable amygdala and were therefore disposed to become inhibited, and which were born with a less excitable amygdala and were therefore disposed to be uninhibited. I now describe these procedures.

Methods

At 2 and 4 months of age, 102 infants were observed in our laboratory while heart rate was recorded across a series of episodes and behavior recorded on audiovisual tape. The first episode was always a 60-second quiet baseline period, followed by a presentation of stimulus episodes from different modalities, and ending with a final baseline. Because we concentrate on the 4-month data in this report, that protocol is now described.

Following the initial baseline period, the infant was presented with four trials of a visual procedure. For each trial the infant was first shown a single three-dimensional stimulus for 10 seconds, followed by a 10-second interstimulus interval, and then a pair of stimuli for 10 seconds. One member of the pair was the object seen earlier, and the other member was a new form of similar size. This procedure was followed by the presentation of three mobiles, varying in the number of elements (one, three, or seven). Each of the three mobiles was presented three times for a total of nine trials, each trial 20 seconds in duration. Following the mobiles the child listened to a tape recording of three syllables spoken by a female voice—"ma," "pa," and "ga"—at three levels of loudness for 12-second durations and a total of nine trials. The child was then presented with a second set of four trials of visual stimulation using the same procedure described earlier for the first visual episode. This procedure was followed by a final baseline period.

At 9 and 14 months of age, the child was observed in three settings—two different small laboratory rooms and a large playroom—in order to assess the propensity to exhibit inhibited or uninhibited behavior. The protocol at 9 months of age follows. Initially, the child and mother came to a small laboratory room for 5 minutes in order to acclimate the child to the room. The examiner then entered and applied electrodes for the recording of heart rate. There was then a baseline period in which the child sat quietly,

followed by an administration of a variation on the object perm-
anence procedure. The mother then took the examiner's seat across
from the child and presented a moving toy dinosaur. During the
first presentation, the mother was instructed to smile but not talk.
During the second presentation, she was instructed to frown. It
was anticipated that the unexpected appearance of the frown on
the mother's face would elicit fear in some children.

The child was then taken to an adjoining room for two procedures. In the first, a bank of colored lights began to flicker on the
right side of the child's visual field; a few seconds later, the lights
went off, and on the left side of the visual field a toy drummer was
activated. This procedure was repeated for seven trials. In the next
procedure, two small puppet heads were presented in an alternating
procedure on the right and left side. One puppet head was painted
with a smile and the second with a frown. As each puppet appeared,
the child heard the tape of a female voice speaking a nonsense
phrase in either a happy or an angry voice. The smiling puppet
was associated with a happy voice and the frowning puppet with
an angry voice. This procedure was repeated for 10 trials.

The child was then taken back to the original room for the final
part of the battery. In the next procedure, a small toy car ran down
an incline for 11 trials. On the early trials it knocked down a tower
of blocks; on the later trials it did not. In the next procedure, the
examiner uncovered a rotating object, and when the child reached
for it, or after a fixed period, the examiner spoke a nonsense
phrase in a happy voice for two trials. On the succeeding two trials
a different toy was presented, but this time the examiner spoke
in an angry, stern voice, supported by a frowning face. The
child was then asked to sit quietly for a quiet baseline, after which
an unfamiliar stranger entered the room and approached the
child.

The electrodes were then removed, and the child and mother
were taken to a large playroom on another floor. For the first 5
minutes the child played while the mother sat on a nearby couch.
An unfamiliar woman then entered, sat down, and remained quiet
for 1 minute. She then began to play with a toy she had brought
for 1 minute, then talked for 1 minute, and finally invited the child
to play. If the child approached the stranger early in the sequence,
the stranger began to play and talk with the child. The stranger
then left, and a mobile car, which was radio-operated from an
adjoining room, began to move in an unpredictable pattern for a 2-

minute period. Finally, the examiner entered and asked the mother to leave the room for a brief period of separation, in which the child was left alone.

The battery administered at 14 months of age was a little different from the one administered at 9 months. The initial warm-up session, application of electrodes, and baseline were the same as described for 9 months. In the next episode, a metal wheel (resembling an open bingo wheel) was rotated by the examiner at three different speeds, each for 10 seconds for six trials. On the first trial the wheel was empty. On the second trial soft cloth objects that made no noise were placed in the wheel. For the next three trials objects that made noise were added in increasing numbers, so that by Trial 5 the wheel made a great deal of noise as it rotated. On the final trial all of the objects were removed, and the wheel was once again silent as it rotated. The child's blood pressure was then taken, both sitting and standing. The child was then asked to imitate the examiner, who implemented six different acts, some of which were unusual (e.g., placing a finger in the open mouth of a large dragonlike animal; putting a hand in black liquid). In the next procedure, the child was requested to taste first sweet and then sour substances from an eyedropper. The child was then presented with the same procedure used at 9 months in which the examiner uncovered a toy and first showed a happy face on two trials and then an angry face. A baseline period was followed by a stranger's entering the room and approaching the child. Finally, the child was taken to the other small laboratory room and shown the puppet procedure, as described at 9 months.

The electrodes were then removed and the child and mother taken to the same large playroom used at 9 months. The first 5 minutes were devoted to free play with the mother, as implemented at 9 months. The woman then rose, went to a corner of the room, opened a cabinet, and uncovered a metal robot about 2.5 feet tall. Initially the woman was quiet for 1 minute and then invited the child to play with the robot while she pressed an electric switch that made the head of the robot light up. At the end of the minute she activated a tape recorder so that a voice appeared to come from the robot. The examiner then left, leaving the child for a final free-play period of 5 minutes. The examiner then returned and asked the mother to leave the child alone for a brief separation period.

Results

One of the obvious differences among the 4-month-old infants involves motor behavior to the stimuli. Some infants were highly aroused motorically; some were minimally aroused. Because we assume that the mechanisms mediating motor arousal do no lie on a continuum, we performed two types of analyses. In the first, two coders independently assigned each infant to a discrete qualitative category of motor arousal, based on the frequency and intensity of limb movements, tongue protrusions, and arches of the back, and an obvious muscular tension and spasticity in the hands and fingers. The amount of vocalization was not used in this classification. The agreement between two coders was high. In addition, a set of different coders performed quantitative analyses by coding the frequency of appearance of limb movements, tongue protrusions, and arches of the back but did not judge the more subtle qualities of motor tension in hands, fingers, and trunk. The correlation between this quantitative index and the categorical judgments was also high.

About 15% of the infants observed were assigned to the category of very high motor arousal and about 20% to a very low motor arousal group. Forty percent of the children were assigned to a category of moderate motor arousal and 25% to a group characterized by moderately high motor arousal. Thus, about 60% of the infants were judged to be low or moderately low in motor arousal, and 40% were judged to be very high or moderately high on motor arousal.

The infants' crying displayed a different distribution. Most children cried very little or not at all. But about one third cried to two or more episodes, and they were called *high criers*. The child's heart rate while sitting quietly was a third variable, which was divided at the mean value, depending upon the sex of the child, for boys have lower heart rates than girls at all ages. Thus, each child could be put into a conjunctive category described by three factors—motor arousal, crying, and heart rate. It should be noted that motor arousal was greater at 2 months than at 4 months, whereas crying was less frequent at the older age. Second, the 4-month behavioral data were better predictors of inhibited and uninhibited behavior later in the year than the behavior at 2 months. However, other aspects of the 2-month performance, especially excessive crying, were predictive of later temperamental style.

The evaluations of the 94 infants seen at both 9 and 14 months contained many occasions on which a child could display obvious signs of fear. As noted in the methods section, there were 14 episodes at 9 months in which the child could meet our criterion for fear—11 in the two small laboratory rooms with the examiner and 3 in the large playroom. At 14 months of age, there were 15 episodes that could be coded for fear—11 in the small laboratory rooms with the examiner and 4 in the large playroom. The main operational definitions of fear in the small laboratory rooms included (a) sudden fretting or crying to application of the electrodes or the blood pressure cuff, to a change of location, to the entrance of the stranger in the small laboratory room, or to a trial of a stimulus episode; (b) reluctance to imitate any of the acts in the episode presented in the 14-month battery or resistance to accept the liquids in the taste episode, accompanied by fretting; (c) in the playroom, retreat to the mother when the stranger entered, accompanied by failure to approach the stranger; (d) failure to approach the robot; or (e) crying to the movements of the radio-controlled car. We did not include distress to separation in our index of fear because we wanted to determine the relation between separation fear and the predisposition to display fear in all of the other situations.

Only a small number of situations elicited obvious fear in the infants. Only 4 of the 14 situations at 9 months met our criteria for fear in at least one fourth of the subjects, and 3 situations did not elicit fear in any child. Five of the 15 situations at 14 months elicited fear from at least one fourth of the children, and at least one child showed fear to every situation. Further, at 9 months the maximum proportion of children showing fear to any episode was 36%. (This was the episode in which the mother frowned while showing the child the toy dinosaur.) At 14 months, 61% of the children showed fear to the robot. (They refused to approach the robot despite urging by the woman.) These facts imply a greater propensity to fear at 14 than at 9 months. This fact is not surprising because the maturational changes that are known to occur between 8 and 12 months are accompanied by an increase in fearfulness to both separation from the parent and to strangers. Distress to maternal separation and to strangers are but two members of a general disposition to become fearful to discrepant events (Kagan, 1984).

The obvious signs of fear (e.g., crying to any one of the discrepant trials in the laboratory episodes, retreat from and failure to approach the stranger or the robot) were characteristic of about one-third of the children. The majority, therefore, did not show obvious fear, even though many displayed a wary face and became subdued. We adopted such a strict criterion for coding fear because of our interest in predicting inhibited behavior. Although most children become subdued in reaction to a discrepant event—this phenomenon is universal—we were interested in those children who became so uncertain that they showed a more intense reaction. Thus, the most accurate way to view our results is to appreciate that only 30% of our 9- and 14-month-old children met our strict criteria for fear on two or three episodes. At 9 months, a frown from an adult was the best incentive for fear, whereas at 14 months the best incentive was the combination of an unfamiliar object (the robot) in the context of an unfamiliar person. When the incentive was only an unfamiliar person, only 25% showed fear, but when that person opened up the cabinet and revealed the robot, 60% were reluctant to approach it despite urging by the person.

SEX DIFFERENCES

Although there was a tendency for girls to be more fearful than boys at both 9 and 14 months, these differences were slight and only occurred for some episodes. And, even in those episodes the differences were not statistically significant. The only episode at 9 months that revealed a sex difference was that in which the mother frowned as she displayed the novel toy. At 14 months, 75% of the girls, but only 50% of the boys, refused to approach the robot.

RELATION TO SEPARATION DISTRESS

As noted, we did not include the child's reaction to the mother's leaving the room as one of our indexes of fear because we wanted to see the relation between fear to our episodes and distress to separation. There was a significant relation for girls between fearfulness to the laboratory events and degree of distress to separation from the mother. Among the 13 girls who displayed a strong reaction to separation at 9 months, 10 were highly fearful and not one was fearless. Among the 15 boys who displayed a strong reaction to separation, 5 were highly fearful and only 2 were fearless in the prior laboratory contexts (see Table 4.1).

TABLE 4.1. Relation of degree of distress to separation and number of fears displayed at 9 months.

Number of fears	No Reaction		Mild to moderate reaction		Strong reaction	
	Boys	Girls	Boys	Girls	Boys	Cirls
0	9	7	3	7	2	0
1	4	3	1	2	1	2
2	4	1	3	5	7	1
≧3	6	6	6	3	5	10

	Sexes pooled		
Number of fears	No reaction	Mild to moderate reaction	Strong reaction
0	16	10	2
1–2	12	11	11
≧3	12	9	15

Thus, the relation between propensity to fearfulness and sep-aration to stress was asymmetrical. Among the 9-month-old chil-dren who did not fret or cry to separation, there were both fearful and nonfearful children. But among the 28 children who reacted with extreme distress, 15 showed high fear to the prior discrepant episodes and 2 were not at all fearful. Thus, an extreme distress reaction to watching the mother leave the room is most character-istic of children who have a general propensity to be fearful of unfamiliar events when the mother is sitting close to them. Because children who show a strong distress reaction are harder to soothe and often resist the mother upon reunion, these data imply a temperamental contribution to the classification called Type C insecure attachment.

There was stability of fear from 9 to 14 months ($r = .44$, $p < .001$). Further, the infants who were classified as high motor-cry-heart rate at 4 months had higher fear scores at both 9 and 14 months than the group classified as low motor-cry-heart rate. However, motor activity and crying were more sensitive predictors of fear; baseline heart rate made a smaller contribution to later fear.

The data in Table 4.2 reveal that only 14 of the 94 children seen at 14 months were high on motor arousal, crying, and fear—about 15% of the sample. This proportion is extremely close to our es-timate of the proportion of inhibited children in the population.

TABLE 4.2. Relation between characteristics of 4-month-old infants and fear behavior at 14 months*.

	Number of fears at 14 months		
	0–1	2–3	≧4
High on motor-cry	1	7	14
Low on motor-cry	20	11	4

* $N = 57$.

Twenty children were fearless and showed low motor arousal and low crying, which is close to our estimate of the 25% of the population who are uninhibited.

Discussion

The corpus of data presented is supportive of the theoretical suggestion that the 1 to 2-year-old children we classify as inhibited or uninhibited differ from each other in the early months of life in the excitability of the amygdala and its projections. The basolateral nucleus of the amygdala, which receives processed visual and auditory information, projects to the ventral striatum and ventral pallidum, and thence to the skeletal motor system directly, as well as indirectly through the thalamus and the supplementary motor cortex. It is possible that the tongue protrusions, back arches, and limb movements seen in highly aroused 4-month-olds are mediated by the circuits coming from this nucleus. A low threshold of excitability in this site could be an important factor mediating the high levels of motor activity in some infants.

The central nucleus of the amygdala represents an important origin for activity in the autonomic nervous system and also influences motor-postural tension and crying through projections to the periaqueductal grey. Thus, a low threshold of excitability in the central nucleus could be associated with motor tension, irritability, and sympathetic reactivity. Finally, the basolateral nucleus synapses on the central nucleus; thus, activity in the former affects the excitability of the latter.

For these reasons we suggest that the highly fearful 14-month-olds, many of whom we believe will show the qualities of inhibited behavior in later childhood, were born with low thresholds in the amygdala, whereas the uninhibited children were born with high thresholds in this site. However, we do not conceive of the two temperamental groups as lying on a continuum. We suggest that the neurochemical basis for the high motor arousal and irritability of the inhibited children is not the complement of the neuro-chemical profile that mediates low motor arousal, low crying, low sympathetic activity, and fearlessness. We recognize that, at the moment, this statement rests mainly on intuition. However, one reason for this suggestion is that the two groups differ in other qualities. The uninhibited children smile more often, especially at 2 and 4 months, whereas the future inhibited children show more grimacing of the face at 2 months of age. Second, their body builds are different. The highly aroused, fearful infants are smaller than the uninhibited ones and are more likely to have blue eyes, light complexions, and blonde hair. We are of the opinion that the categories we call inhibited and uninhibited children are analogous to strains of monkeys that differ on a profile of qualities rather than on a single dimension.

Acknowledgment. The research described in this report was supported by a grant from the John D. and Catherine T. MacArthur Foundation.

References

Braverman, N.C. (1989). Physiological profiles of shy and sociable college women. Unpublished senior honors thesis, Harvard-Radcliffe College, Cambridge, MA.

Clarke, A.S., Mason, W.A., & Moberg, J.P. (1988). Differential behavioral and adrenocortical responses to stress among three macaques species. *American Journal of Primatology, 14*, 13–52.

Davidson, R.J., & Fox, N.A. (1989). Frontal brain asymmetry predicts infants' response to maternal separation. *Journal of Abnormal Psychology, 98*, 127–131.

Davidson, R.J., & Tomarken, A.J. (1989). Laterality and emotion: Electro-physiological approach. In F. Boller & J. Grafman (Eds.), *Handbook of Neuropsychology* (Vol. 3, pp. 419–441). Amsterdam: Elsevier.

Eysenck, H.J. (1953). *The structure of human personality.* London: Methuen.

Jung, C.G. (1924). *Psychological types.* New York: Harcourt Brace.

Kagan, J. (1984). *The Nature of the Child.* New York: Basic Books.

LaGasse, L.L., Gruber, C.P., & Lipsitt, L.P. (1989). The infantile expression of avidity in relation to later assessments of inhibition and attachment.

In J.S. Reznick (Ed.), *Perspectives on behavioral inhibition* (pp. 159–176). Chicago: University of Chicago Press.

Schneirla, T.C. (1965). Aspects of stimulation and organization in approach-withdrawal processes in vertebrate development. In D.S. Lehrman, R.A. Hinde, & E. Shaw (Eds.), *Advances in the study of behavior* (Vol. 1, pp. 1–74). New York: Academic Press.

Scott, J.P., & Fuller, J.L. (1965). *Genetics and the social behavior of the dog.* Chicago: University of Chicago Press.

5
The Challenge Facing Infant Research in the Next Decade[1]

Frances Degen Horowitz

In January of 1990, the *Merrill-Palmer Quarterly* published a special issue devoted to the topic of infancy. It contained a set of papers written by some of the most senior infant researchers—each summing up a particular area and trying to assess where we have been, what we now know, and what the future agenda in the area is likely to be. This special issue was occasioned by the fact that it was about 20 years ago that the Merrill-Palmer Symposium on Infancy was inaugurated, and it seemed to the editors of the quarterly that it was time to take stock. Many of those invited to contribute to the special issue were among the early participants in the Merrill-Palmer symposium and in the general revival of infant research that occurred in the 1960s.

The decade of the 60s and the years in the 70s to follow can be thought of as quite heady times for child development in general and for the study of infancy in particular. I have referred to many of the infant studies of those years as representatives of a kind of "gee whiz" science: Gee whiz—look at what babies can do that we never thought them capable of. See—here is the newborn baby who responds discriminatively in every sensory modality (Clifton, Graham, & Hatton, 1968; Fantz, 1958; Friedman, 1972; Self, Horowitz, & Paden, 1972; Stechler, Bradford, & Levy, 1966); here is the newborn infant whose behavior can be conditioned

---

[1] This chapter was written during the author's tenure at the University of Kansas, Lawrence, KS.

(Siqueland & Lipsitt, 1966); here are infants at birth and in the first year of life demonstrating surprising and interesting abilities— abilities that led Stone and his colleagues to publish, in 1973, their book entitled *The Competnet Infant* (Stone, Smith, & Murphy, 1973). In that year, also, was the first edition of the Neonatal Behavioral Assessment Scale (Brazelton, 1973). Within 5 years we have the founding of the journal *Infant Behavior and Development* and the International Conference on Infancy Studies. And it all continued unabated into the 80s. *Infant Behavior and Development* has been complemented by a monograph series, and there is not a single issue of all the major child development journals that does not contain one or more, sometimes many, reports on infant behavior and development.

Amid this outpouring of facts, it is almost curious that theory has been essentially nonexistent. Though one might have expected that the initial flurry of infant conditioning studies in the 1960s and more recently would have contributed to the development of learning theory and to behaviorism in general, such has not been the case. The role of Piaget's theory in stimulating some of the first studies of infant perception and cognition in the 1960s might have been thought to have made important contributions to Piagetian theory. Instead, as the phenomena studied turned out to be somewhat less regular than Piaget's theory predicted but more interesting in their own right, less and less attention has been directed toward the theory itself and more to exploring infant behaviors and the manner in which they function.

A similar picture emerges when one thinks about the relevance of psychodynamic and Freudian theory in the context of studies of attachment and, more recently, emotional development. Yet here, too, the focus has been not so much upon the theoretical import of the evidence but upon the facts themselves. Whole areas of infant research commanding large amounts of resources and significant numbers of investigators, such as risk and high-risk infant research, have been largely atheoretical. Parke (1989), in his discussion of social development, notes that this field has been marked by the prevalence of minitheories and more domain-specific theory, but the facts remain largely unintegrated.

Such a state of affairs, it seems to me, presents a major challenge to the field of infant research, and it is this challenge and its various dimensions that I would like to explore in this chapter. In addressing this challenge I intend to focus on the following issues and questions: Is infancy a special period? How is research in infancy best related to questions of continuity and discontinuity and to the heredity/environment controversy? Are there recent developments that require us to readjust the focus of our inquiries? And, finally, are there recent theoretical developments that are more than minitheory possibilities?

Is Infancy a Special Period?

We all know that infancy is a period of rapid development with significant amounts of regularity from individual to individual. For this reason some believe infancy is a more evolutionarily buffered period than other periods of development. The basic species' typical patterns of development are seen as under the control of genetic and biological factors to such a degree that differential environmental impact on development during infancy is thought to be negligible (Kagan, Kearsley, & Zelazo, 1978; Scarr-Salapatek, 1976). From this position one expects environmental variations to have relatively little lasting effect on subsequent developmental outcome. It would follow, then, that the principal task of researchers interested in infants would be to document the basic patterns of behavior and to investigate individual differences on the assumption that they are biologically and genetically determined.

On the other hand, we have a quite contrary set of beliefs wherein infancy is required as a special period just because variations in environmental experience have a greater and more lasting impact than is true for other periods of development. This point of view found support in Hebb's theory of the role of environmental stimulation on early development (Hebb, 1949) and in the classic chapter by Sameroff and Chandler (1975), in which they proposed that the effects of adverse prenatal and perinatal factors on developmental outcome were mediated by the nature of environmental experience during the postnatal period. Greater brain plasticity in infancy leaves more room for environmental impact. Much of the intervention research with high-risk populations of infants is premised on the belief that early intervention and/or stimulation, appropriately administered, can have significant effect on developmental outcome (Horowitz, 1980, 1989b; Horowitz & Paden, 1973).

One strategy for reconciling these two seemingly incompatible positions is to consider both of them partially correct. As I have suggested elsewhere (Horowitz, 1987), it is not unreasonable to propose the obvious: Namely, the human behavioral repertoire contains behaviors that are species-typical and thus universal; the human behavioral repertoire is also made up of behaviors that are not universal. These behaviors are culturally determined and environmentally fostered, though many of the nonuniversal behaviors may be based or built upon one or more of the universal behaviors.

Such an ecumenical strategy does not, however, fully address the question of whether infancy is a special period. In order to retain the notion that infancy has particular characteristics not shared by other periods of development, one would have to maintain that the rate of density of development of universal behaviors is greater during infancy than during other developmental periods. And one would have to pose the question of whether or not environmental impact is in any way different or more permanent when it occurs during infancy as compared to environmental effects at other periods of development.

Continuity, Discontinuity, or Both?

This last comment, of course, raises the next question. What light is shed on the questions of continuity and discontinuity in development from our understanding of development during infancy? Almost the entirety of a recent issue of *Human Development* was given over to the discussion of continuity and discontinuity (*Human Development*, 1989, 3–4). As well, numerous chapters have appeared recently on this topic (e.g., Rutter, 1987). We are actually in a period of considerable ferment in relation to the question of whether development is best thought of in terms of continuities or discontinuities.

What is swirling about us are data from a number of sources. First, there is the assessment of visual habituation and novelty preference showing some prediction to later IQ (Fagan & Singer, 1983; Rose, Feldman, Wallace, & McCarton, 1989; Slater, Cooper, Roser, & Morison, 1989; Bornstein, 1989). However, the amount of variance accounted for by these predictions generally does not exceed what we can already account for by parental education (McCall, 1989, 1990), though there is the puzzling aspect that parental education and novelty recognition do not appear, them-selves, to be correlated. The degree of prediction is variable among different populations, and there is the further problem that the day-to-day reliabilities and even problem-to-problem reliabilities in the novelty recognition and habituation tasks are not particularly high. How do these data address the question of whether we have continuity or discontinuity from infancy to later childhood in rela-tion to early cognitive and later IQ?

Second, there are the data from various studies of attachment that show evidence of some continuity across time in individual differences (Sroufe & Jacobvitz, 1989). Additionally, as we have seen today, there is some prediction from individual difference characteristics such as being inhibited and noninhibited (see Chapter 4 by Kagan & Snidman, this volume). Yet there is plenty of room for discontinuity. Indeed, Baumrind (1989) contends that we ought to expect development to be basically discontinuous since development means change.

Alternatively, and more to the commonsense side of things, it may be best to characterize development as both continuous and discontinuous (e.g., Sternberg & Okagaki, 1989). Might we, for example, expect continuity to be more characteristic of those behaviors that are universals but bounded by particular individual difference characteristics that are biologically or genetically based? And might we also expect discontinuity in those behaviors that are most influenced by environmental impact when the nature of the environmental conditions change over time, whereas if the en-vironmental conditions remain stable we will see continuity? For example, achievement in school may be highly impacted by sup-portive environmental conditions. If the environment becomes nonsupportive, achievement levels may be discontinuous; if they remain supportive, achievement levels will show stability (i.e., continuity).

Much of the continuity/discontinuity discussion has focused on particular developmental phenomena such as IQ, attachment, or personality characteristics. A somewhat different approach to the continuity/discontinuity question would be to ask not whether a particular characteristic shows continuity or discontinuity but whether the processes involved in a developmental domain show continuity or discontinuity (Horowitz, 1987). As we shall see later in this discussion, framing the question in this manner would result in a quite different set of developmental research strategies.

To what extent is the period of infancy particularly relevant to the understanding of continuity and discontinuity in development? If, in fact, the majority of the behaviors that develop during the period of infancy are of the universal kind, would we expect more continuity in these behaviors from infancy to later periods of development? On the other hand, suppose infancy is an evolutionarily buffered period with less sensitivity to environmental variations. Then we would expect less continuity from infancy to later periods because at these later periods we would have the contribution of environmental effects on development that introduce factors and amounts of variance that were not present at the earliest developmental period.

Heredity and/or Environment?

This brings us to the most classic of all questions: Heredity or environment, or both? The earliest environmental interventions were aimed at trying to answer this question (see Skeels, 1966), though few of these efforts involved any measure of heredity or genes and their contributions. More recently, of course, the field of behavior genetics, with a host of sophisticated indirect measures of genetic influence, has produced impressive data that permit the inference of genetic contributions to observed variance in the domains of intellectual and social behavior and personality characteristics (Plomin, 1986, 1989).

On the environmental side, we have all the intervention efforts aimed at various high-risk populations, some of which have known genetic defects. For example, there are the interventions with Down's syndrome infants, who show a significant developmental progress as a function of the intervention and higher levels of developmental outcome than would otherwise be expected (Bricker, 1982). Most of the intervention efforts with infants have involved those whose socioeconomic backgrounds put them at social risk, though it is assumed that soft biological risks are present as correlates of social risk conditions. Disentangling the genetic and environmental contributions in these studies has been difficult (Garber, 1988; Garber & Hodge, 1989; Jensen, 1989). Further, it is not always clear whether the term *constitutional* is synonymous with *genetic*. For example, fetal alcohol syndrome produces constitutional defects that are not genetic defects. On the other hand, there are genetic defects that are functionally synonymous with constitutional defects.

I am fond of pointing out that the only purely genetic moment in the history of an organism is at conception. Between conception and birth one has the playing out of genes and their influences in the context of a prenatal environment that affects genes and that affects the biological functioning of the organism. This may seem to some a subtle distinction, but it is an important one, whether or not one buys into Susan Oyama's insistence that there is no genetic program but only genes that develop in and as a function of environment (Oyama, 1985). Because the cumulated amount of time for environmental influence to be at work is briefer for infants, would we expect a greater influence of genetic and constitutional variables to be in evidence during this period? A recent report by Loehlin and his colleagues (Loehlin, Horn, & Willerman, 1989) suggests that genetic influences do not necessarily evidence themselves once and for all time during infancy, after which all further variables are based in the environment. Rather, they reported that although genes and family environment variables contributed to a measure of intellectual function at a first test, only inferred genetic variance made an additional contribution at a later test time. The subjects in the Loehlin et al. study varied widely in age at first testing, so the point being made here is not specific to infancy, though the possibility of differential impact of genetic and environmental variables across the life span is of some relevance. It must be noted, however, that many of the behavior genetic studies involve adopted children. Little is known about differential environments provided by the same parents for adopted as compared with biological children. It is assumed that adopted and biological children reared together have a commonly shared family environment, but this assumption bears some investigation. If there is anything to the possibility of matched and mismatched parents and children and differential environmental contexts, it is also possible that parents have a higher chance of mismatch with their adopted children in comparison with their biological children.

None of this should be taken in any way to suggest that genes and genetic variance are not relevant to understanding behavioral development. Nor should it be used to dismiss genetic and nongenetic constitutional influences. However, what is being suggested is that a more complex and sophisticated model of development may be necessary to our current discourse than is implied in a question about the influence of heredity and/or environment. And this complex model ought to be able to address the issue of whether or not infancy as a period of development has any particular aspects that distinguish it from other periods of development.

Recent Developments and an Adjusted Focus?

Though behavior genetics has probably had the most impact on the consideration of heredity and environmental influences on development, there are other recent developments that have a much greater potential for influencing how we look at development and developmental processes. As Kendler (1989) has noted, because behaviorism eschewed inclusion in a scientific account of any variables for which measurement was not possible, in the years before reliable measures of internal variables were available, behaviorists could be thought of as assuming an "empty organism." Today, as a result of major advances in the neurosciences, such measures are increasingly available. In addition to the imaging of brain structure, we can now image brain function; we have many more, and more sensitive, tests for measures of physiological function.

The speculations of the cognitivists and the organismic orientations can now be replaced by actual measures of organic function and state. This all requires what I have called a new frame for our science. The new frame essentially makes the old behaviorist/cognitivist argument and dialogue obsolete (Horowitz, 1989a). The implications here are manifold. It has especial importance for understanding development during infancy because of the possibilities that are opened up with respect to measures of variables that influence prenatal development, to measures of neurological function correlates of learning, of cognition, and of perception in a variety of sensory domains. These kinds of physiological measures, some of which are discussed in this volume, give us a window into the organic level that we have not had before. Analog animal studies that trace the neural pathways for the effects of cognitive and emotional experiences are making it possible to ask questions about propositions as diverse as Freudian claims for the primacy of early emotional experience and the neural consequences of learning and perception.

Among the most exciting possibilities with respect to studying infant behavior and development are efforts to understand brain function and development during this period and to investigate the possible two-way street of influence—brain mechanisms that control the nature of the effect of environmental input and brain mechanisms that are affected by environmental input. We are not dealing here with the simple possibilities of reductionism but rather with dynamic interactions more complex than we have previously thought possible. Organismic variables have been made exceedingly more visible through direct measurement.

Although the measurement of organismic variables has improved significantly, we cannot say the same about progress with respect to defining environmental variables and to refining our measurement of these variables. We need much more attention to the question of what the functional units of environmental variables are. This is of particular importance to those who are interested in infants because not only is the infant organism highly dependent for its survival on environmental variables but some environmental variables also play a large role in mediating other environmental variables—for example, caretakers who control some aspects of environmental experience. Wachs (1989, 1990) and his colleagues have been making some efforts in this direction, but it is not clear how successful they will be. Though we have more environmental measures available than ever before, ranging from the HOME scale to all manner of environmental observational coding schemes, there is no functionally based system of environmental measures that is rooted in either theory or strong empirical relationships. Because infants are more dependent upon environmental context than is true for older children, serious and systematic attention to the question of the functional units of environment are especially relevant for understanding the impact of environment during infancy—if, in fact one agrees to the notion that infancy is a period during which environment makes a difference.

The Question of Theory

Having said all of this, let us turn to the challenge of theory and theory building as it is related to infancy and to development in general. I believe that the explosion of facts has positioned us very well to return to issues of theory—not minitheory and domain-specific theory, but an overarching view of the elements that contribute to behavioral development and how they may be organized. I would like to suggest the complexity that I believe developmental

TABLE 5.1. Theoretical propositions about behavioral development.

1. Developmental outcome is best described by an equation involving a set of
   variables with given weights and interactive relationships.
2. The same outcome can result from different developmental pathways.
3. The nature of the equation, the variables and their weighting is not necessarily
   the same for each domain or for each period of development.
4. Universal behaviors in their general topography are less influenced by variations
   in the environment than are the nonuniversal behaviors, though
   environmental variations affect the "quality" of universal behaviors as well as
   nonuniversal behaviors.

theory must now encompass. Four propositions (shown in Table
5.1) describe my perspective.

First, I believe that developmental outcome at any point in time
is best described by an equation that involves a set of variables
with given weights and interactive relationships. Second, I believe,
in line with many of the assumptions of systems theory (von
Bertalanffy, 1968), that the same outcome can occur as a result of
different pathways (or different equations) (Sroufe & Jacobvitz,
1989). Third, the nature of the equation, the variables, and their
weightings are not necessarily the same for each domain of development or for each period of development. Fourth, the distinction
between universals and nonuniversals in behavior has important
implications for processes and how they function in the developmental equation. Universal behaviors in their general topography
will be less influenced by variations in environment than nonuniversal behaviors. Learning, culture, and variations in environmental experience and organismically based variables are
relevant to the quality of the universal behaviors, if not the general
topography. The dimensions relevant to the acquisition of nonuniversal behaviors include organismically based individual
differences as well as learning and the organization of the environment, including what is made more or less salient by culture. (See
Horowitz, 1987, for full discussion of these issues.)

The challenge for developmentalists is to begin to formulate the
nature of these equations for different periods of development and
for different domains. We can visualize a set of simultaneous
equations for different domains. Such a possibility suggests that
there are equational interactions that exert control over development. Thelen's (1989) discussion of dynamical systems theory is

relevant here. Her formulation, in the tradition of systems theory, places development within an environmental context, though it is not clear where and how she factors in environmental variations in the dynamic relationships.

An example of the simultaneous equation strategy during infancy may be helpful. Brain plasticity and environmental stimulation may be the significant variables in the acquisition of the non-universal aspects of language development. This may be especially the case for those aspects of language acquisition that depend upon individual differences in sensitivity to environmental input and opportunities for learning. Motor development may, at the same time, be most influenced by organismic variables that are strongly vectored along the lines of speciestypical developmental patterns. On the other hand, brain plasticity may be less of a variable in language acquisition at later ages, though there may be some later developmental periods when it reemerges as an important factor. Constitutionally based individual differences may contribute to some domains more than others. Some constitutionally based variables may only carry important weight in the equation when they take the more extreme values for particular individuals. Or, they may be particularly important during one period of development.

It does not take much to see the combinations and permutations of such complex sets of equations. One of the important implications here is that our goal should be to focus on the processes of development and not the products. If the products of development can occur from development that proceeds along a variety of pathways, by attending to the products or results we will never understand the processes. The issue, therefore, is not continuity or discontinuity of intelligence, personality, or social behavior—or of learning strategies. Rather, it is a matter of knowing the processes responsible for the behaviors in each of these domains and tracking whether the process changes or does not change and whether, as a result, one sees continuity or discontinuity.

Concluding Comments

In conclusion, one can say that the challenge facing infant research in the next decade has several aspects. One is to begin to try to formulate theory that has some chance of accounting for the plethora of interesting facts we now have about infant behavior development. A second aspect of the challenge is to formulate theory that can be used to address the question of what variables— to what degree and in what combination—distinguish infancy from other periods of development. A third part of the challenge is to refocus the questions so that we are concerned about process and not about continuity and discontinuity per se or about heredity and environment per se. And fourth and finally, the challenge is, as always, to use our knowledge in its current state as wisely as possible. Children cannot wait to grow up until we know all we need to know to help them. We must apply our knowledge in its most imperfect state. However, in doing so, we must be careful not to give the false impression of a certainty we do not have. The media are ever hungry to announce our latest findings. In co-operating with this desire, it is incumbent upon each of us to qualify our statements to the fullest. That, of course, will make the media uninterested in us.

Last of all I wish to note that it has fallen to me to close this symposium that honors the career of our colleague Henry Ricciuti. Henry is honored if only by the range of topics represented here today—topics in which he has had an interest and areas to which he has made some contributions. If each of us, in our contributions to this book and in our continuing work, has and continues to aspire to the standards that Henry Ricciuti's work exemplifies we shall, in addition to our writings here, continue to honor him.

References

Baumrind, D. (1989). The performance of change and the impermanence of stability. *Human Development, 32,* 187–195.

Bornstein, M.H. (1989). Information processing (habituation) in infancy and stability in cognitive development. *Human Development, 32,* 129–136.

Brazelton, T.B. (1973). *The neonatal behavioral assessment scale* (1st ed.). Philadelphia: Lippincott.

Bricker, D. (1982). Program planning for at-risk and handicapped infants. In C.T. Ramey & P.L. Trhoanis (Eds.), *Finding and educating high risk and handicapped infants* (pp. 119–135). Baltimore; MD: University Park Press.

Clifton, R.K., Graham, F.K., & Hatton, H.M. (1968). Newborn heart rate response and response habituation as a function of stimulus duration. *Journal of Experimental Child Psychology, 6,* 265–278.

Fagan, J.F., & Singer, L.T. (1983). Infant recognition memory as a measure of intelligence. In L.P. Lipsitt & C.K. Rovee-Collier (Eds.), *Advances in infancy research* (pp. 31–78). Norwood, NJ: Ablex Publishing Corporation.

Fantz, R. (1958). Pattern vision in young infants. *Psychological Record, 8,* 43–47.

Friedman, S. (1972). Newborn visual attention to repeated exposure of redundant vs. "novel" targets. *Perception and Psychophysics,12,* 291–294.

Garber, H.L. (1988). *The Milwaukee project.* Washington, DC: American Association on Mental Retardation.

Garber, H.L., & Hodge, J.D. (1989). Reply: Risk for deceleration in rate of mental development. *Developmental Review, 9,* 259–300.

Hebb, D.O. (1949). *The organization of behavior.* New York: Wiley.

Horowitz, F.D. (1980). Intervention and its effects of early development: What model of development is appropriate? In R. Turner & H.W. Reese (Eds.), *Life span development psychology intervention* (pp.235–248). New York: Academic Press, 235–248.

Horowitz, F.D. (1987). *Exploring developmental theories: Toward a structural/ behavioral model of development.* Hillsdale, NJ: Erlbaum. Horowitz, F.D. (1989a). *On the nature of dialogues in the behavioral sciences.* Unpublished paper to the Department of Human Development and Family Life at the University of Kansas.

Horowitz, F.D. (1989b). Using developmental theory to guide the search for the effects of biological risk factors of the development of children. *Journal of Clinical Nutrition, 50,* 589–597.

Horowitz, F.D., & Paden, L.Y. (1973). The effectiveness of environmental intervention programs. In B.M. Caldwell & H.N. Ricciuti (Eds.), *Review of child development research* (Vol. 3, pp. 331–402). Chicago: University of Chicago Press. *Human Development.* (1989). 3–4.

Jensen, A.R. (1989). Raising IQ without increasing *g*? A review of "The Milwaukee project: Preventing mental retardation in children at risk." *Developmental Review, 9,* 234–258.

Kagan, J., Kearsley, R.B., & Zelazo, P.R. (1978). *Infancy.* Cambridge, MA: Harvard University Press.

Kendler, H.H. (1989). The Iowa tradition. *American Psychologist, 44,* 1124–1132.

Loehlin, J.C., Horn, J.M., & Willerman, L. (1989). Modeling IQ change: Evidence from the Texas Adoption Project. *Child Development, 60,* 993–1004.

McCall, R.B. (1989). Issues in predicting later IQ from infant habituation rate and recognition memory performance. *Human Development, 32,* 177–186.

MacCall, R.B. (1990). Infancy research: Individual differences. *Merrill-Palmer Quarterly, 36,* 141–158.

Oyama, S. (1985). *The ontogeny of information.* Cambridge: Cambridge University Press.

Parke, R.D. (1989). Social development in infancy: A 25-year perspective. In H.W. Reese (Ed.), *Advances in child development and behavior* (pp. 1–48). New York: Academic Press.

Plomin, R. (1986). *Development, genetics and psychology*. Hillsdale, NJ: Erlbaum.

Plomin, R. (1989). Environment and genes: Determinants of behavior. *American Psychologist*.

Rose, S.A., Feldman, J.F., Wallace, I.F., & McCarton, C. (1989). Infant visual attention: Relation to birth status and developmental outcome during the first 5 years. *Developmental Psychology, 25,* 560–576.

Rutter, M. (1987). Continuities and discontinuities for infancy. In J.D. Osofsky (Ed.), *Handbook of infant development* (2nd ed., pp. 1256–1296). New York: Wiley and Sons.

Sameroff, A.J., & Chandler, M.J. (1975). Reproductive risk and the continuum of caretaking casualty. In F.D. Horowitz (Ed.), *Review of child development research* (Vol. 4, pp. 187–244). Chicago: University of Chicago Press.

Scarr-Salapatek, S. (1976). An evolutionary perspective on infant intelligence. In M. Lewis (Ed.), *Origins of intelligence: Infancy and early childhood* (pp. 165–197). New York: Plenum.

Self, P., Horowitz, F.D., & Paden, L.Y. (1972). Olfaction in newborn infants. *Developmental Psychology, 7,* 349–363.

Siqueland, E.R., & Lipsitt, L.P. (1966). Conditioned head-turning behavior in newborns. *Journal of Experimental Child Psychology, 3,* 356–376.

Skeels, H.M. (1966). Adult status of children with contrasting early life experiences: A follow-up study. *Monographs of the Society for Research in Child Development, 31*(Serial No. 105).

Slater, A., Cooper, R., Rose, D., & Morison, V. (1989). Prediction of cognitive performance from infancy to early childhood. *Human Development, 32,* 137–147.

Sroufe, L.A., & Jacobvitz, D. (1989). Diverging pathways, developmental transformations, multiple etiologies and the problem of continuity in development. *Human Development, 32,* 196–203.

Stechler, G., Bradford, S., & Levy, H. (1966). Attention in the newborn: Effect on motility and skin potential. *Science, 151,* 1247–1248.

Sternberg, R.J., & Okagaki, L. (1989). Continuity and discontinuity in intellectual development are not a matter of "either-or." *Human Development, 32,* 158–166.

Stone, J., Smith, H., & Murphy, L. (Eds.). (1973). *The competent infant*. New York: Basic Books.

Thelen, E. (1989). Self-organization in developmental processes: Can systems approaches work? In M.R. Gunnar & E. Thelen (Eds.), *Systems and development Minnesota symposia on child psychology* (Vol. 22, pp.77–117). Hillsdale, NJ: Erlbaum.

von Bertalanffy, L. (1968). *General system theory* (rev. ed.). New York George Braziller.

Wachs, T.D. (1989). The nature of the physical environment: An expanded classification system. *Merrill-Palmer Quarterly, 35,* 399–420.

Wachs, T.D. (1990). Must the physical environment be mediated by the social environment in order to influence development?: A further test. *Journal of Applied Developmental Psychology, 11,* 163–178.

6

Current and Future Directions in Infant Development Research: Brief Overview

Henry N. Ricciuti

This chapter presents a brief summary of what I perceive to be some of the most significant areas of emphasis that characterize contemporary research on infant behavior and development, and that are also likely to represent future directions of very active and productive inquiry. Some of these areas of emphasis are clearly illustrated in the empirical research reported in the present book's chapters by Kagan and Snidman (Chapter 4), Osofsky and Eberhard-Wright (Chapter 2), and Pollitt, Gorman, and Metallinos-Katsaras (Chapter 3), while several areas have already been alluded to in the review chapters by Parke (Chapter 1) and Horowitz (Chapter 5).

As pointed out in both Parke's and Horowitz's chapters, the field of infant research has grown tremendously over the past 30 years or so, and it continues to flourish with great vigor. One of the reasons for this continued growth is the fact that many of the issues addressed by infant researchers represent problems that are of broad significance in the study of human development and are not limited in their relevance only to the first few years of life. The brief overview presented below identifies some of these major research trends, which are viewed as representing naturally evolving shifts in orientation from those characterizing earlier periods of research in this field.

One of the particularly interesting overall trends, apparent across most areas of infant research, is the simultaneous emergence of significantly increased and more sophisticated basic research activity, along with an increasing concern with the utilization of research for applied purposes. This application of research has tended to focus particularly on the broad issue of preventing potentially adverse developmental outcomes, as well as optimizing conditions for ensuring that children reach their developmental potential (also mentioned by Parke, Chapter 1, this volume). At the same time, there has been an increasing involvement, at least on the part of many infant researchers, in articulating broad social policy implications of research on infant development. Now let me become a bit more specific.

Increasing Linkages of Behavioral and Biological Perspectives

One of the most important major shifts in emphasis is that represented by the increasing merger of biological and behavioral perspectives in approaching developmental problems (as pointed out by both Parke and Horowitz). These bio-behavioral linkages can take a variety of forms, including the following: (a) increasingly sophisticated studies of the behavioral consequences of a variety of carefully specified prenatal and perinatal risk conditions, such as intraventricular hemorrhages in very low birth weight infants (Sostek, Smith, Katz, & Grant, 1987; Williams, Lewandowski, Coplan, & D'Eugenio, 1983), exposure to prenatal teratogens such as drugs (Jones & Lopez, 1988) or PCB (Jacobson, Fein, Jacobson, Schwartz, & Dowler, 1985), and so forth (see also Kopp & Kaler, 1989); (b) more systematic consideration of the role of brain chemistry in infant behavior and development, for example, the role of brain hormones or neurotransmitters in explaining the potential behavioral effects of early iron deficiency (Evans, 1985; Youdim, Ben-Shachar, & Yehuda, 1989), or the etiology of behavioral differences between inhibited and noninhibited infants and young children (Kagan, this volume), or the nature of infants' affective responses (Fox, 1988); (c) examination of biologically determined regularities and patterns of organization of spontaneous activity in fetal and early postnatal life (Robertson, 1987); (d) exploration of parallels between physical growth and early mental development (Pollitt, this volume; Hack & Breslau, 1986); and (e) analysis of socioenvironmental factors influencing infant health, growth, and development (Tinsley & Holtgrave, 1989), including failure to thrive (Bithoney & Newberger, 1987; Drotar & Eckerle, 1989).

An increasingly recognized important perspective in this area is the view that the influence of biological conditions, or risk factors, can only be understood through their interactions with social and environmental circumstances (Breitmayer & Ramey, 1986; Ricciuti & Scarr, 1990). It is considered essential, therefore, that the nature of such biological-environmental interactions continue to be thoroughly investigated (Ricciuti & Dorman, 1983).

More Precise Specification of Infants' Physical and Social Environments and Their Effects on Development

Paralleling the increasing attention being paid to the influence of biological, or organismic, variables is the continued attention being addressed to the problem of defining developmentally relevant, specific components of the infant's environment. Although such efforts would profit from more systematic, overall theoretical formulations (as pointed out in Horowitz, Chapter 5, this volume), a great deal of progress has been made in defining development-ally salient, specific features of the infant's physical and social environment, both proximal and distal (Gottfried, 1984; Wachs & Gruen, 1982). Examples include recent work on the conceptual-ization and measurement of specific dimensions of the physical environment, (Wachs, 1989), various aspects of quality of care in the home environment (Bradley et al., 1989), and specific features of quality of care provided infants in day-care environments (Phillips, 1987).

A great deal of research effort continues to address the difficult problem of characterizing the day-to-day interactions of infants and their primary caregivers, and the nature of the parent-infant or caregiver-infant relationships that such interactions imply (Hann, 1989). Some of this research takes the form of observational coding of increasingly detailed behaviors as they occur sequentially in ongoing adult-infant interaction (Olson, Bayles, & Bates 1986), whereas other investigators employ procedures for rating quali-tative features of the interaction on carefully defined, summary rating scales (Cox, Owen, Lewis, & Henderson, 1989; McAnarney, Lawrence, Ricciuti, Polley, & Szilagyi, 1986). With both approaches, however, major efforts are being made to move beyond separate measures of adult and infant behavior toward the assessment of characteristics of the dyadic interactions as such (Booth, Lyons, & Barnard, 1984; Cohn & Tronick, 1987). This approach is nicely illustrated in Osofsky and Eberhart-Wright's chapter (Chapter 2) in this book, which describes the approach to measuring characteristics of the mother-infant relationship such as reciprocity and emotional availability.

In dealing with the question of how environments influence infant development, increasing attention is being paid to the role of genetic factors, in both parents and children, which can play a role in shaping the "functional" environment experienced by the child (Plomin, 1989). For example, genetically determined parental characteristics may significantly influence the kind of social and physical environment in which they rear their children (Plomin, Loehlin, & De Fries, 1985). Similarly, characteristics of a particular child may influence how that child selects or interacts with various aspects of a given environment (Scarr & Ricciuti, 1991). At the same time, such individual child characteristics may lead to sub-stantially differential treatment of siblings who live in the same household (Plomin & Daniels, 1987), part of the issue of "non-shared, within-family environmental influences" (McCall, 1983).

Finally, although major emphasis in the approaches just de-scribed has tended to be placed on specifying features of the child's proximal environment or interactions in the home or out-of-home setting, the importance of taking account of the broader social environment or social context in which families live has been increasingly recognized (Bronfenbrenner, 1986). For example, studies continue to document the importance of various kinds of social support and stresses that may impinge on parents and families, thus influencing both parenting behavior as well as developmental outcomes in infants and young children (Belsky, 1984; Crittenden, 1985; Ricciuti & Dorman, 1983).

Long-Term Consequences of Early Experience

Among the oldest problems in developmental psychology, ques-tions having to do with the importance of early experience and of critical periods in development continue to be addressed but with fresh perspectives and more sophisticated conceptual and analytic models. In contrast to widely held earlier views, which emphasized relatively fixed developmental trajectories resulting from biological endowment and from experiences early in life, contemporary approaches tend to be centered on explaining the frequently ob-served plasticity of development (Cocking, 1986), and the resilience or "invulnerability" of many children who appear to overcome adverse early experiences (Anthony & Cohler, 1987; Werner &

Smith, 1982; Werner, 1988; Osofsky & Eberhart-Wright, Chapter 2, this volume). At the same time, as suggested also by Horowitz (Chapter 5, this volume), contemporary investigators recognize the importance of the view that equivalent developmental outcomes may be reached by a variety of different developmental pathways.

Continuing interest in these issues is reflected both in long-term studies of naturally occurring variations in early experience, as well as in the many studies of early intervention aimed at altering children's experiences in the interest of preventing unfavorable outcomes, or of optimizing developmental opportunities. In both instances, it has been increasingly recognized that analysis of the long-term consequences of early experiences requires that the developmental mechanisms and pathways that are operative during the course of development must be more fully understood. A very helpful conceptualization of these processes is represented by the "transactional" view of development, which emphasizes, for example, the need to understand how children and their environments (including parents) may dynamically influence and shape each other over time through the life course (Seifer & Sameroff, 1987). With regard to the question of long-term effects of early intervention, it is precisely because of our limited understanding of such ongoing developmental processes and pathways that the late-appearing, so-called sleeper effects purportedly due to much earlier intervention (Lazar & Darlington, 1982; Rauh, Achenbach, Nurcombe, Howell, & Teti, 1988) cannot yet adequately be explained (Woodhead, 1988).

A related issue that illustrates the heuristic value of a transactional perspective on long-term development has to do with the frequent (and generally rather unsuccessful) efforts of developmentalists to predict children's later intellectual status from developmental assessments made in the first 2 years of life. Several studies suggest that such predictions can be substantially improved if one takes into account the nature of the ongoing or subsequent social environment in which the child is living (Beckwith & Cohen, 1984; Siegel, 1982).

Finally, given the nature of the social changes taking place in our society, it is very likely that research on the long-term developmental effects of early experience will focus increasingly on the influence of such factors as maternal employment (Gottfried & Gottfried, 1988); nonmaternal care (Fein & Fox, 1988; McCartney, 1990); adolescent parenting (Garcia-Coll, Vohr, Hoffman, & Oh,

1986); single parenthood (Allen, Affleck, McGrade, & McQueeney, 1984); and the emerging variations in infant care likely to be associated with joint custody (Wolchik, Braver, & Sandler, 1985) or with parenting by lesbian or gay couples (Pollack & Vaughn, 1987).

Early Identification of Developmental Risk

One of the clearest manifestations of developmentalists' growing concern with utilizing research to enhance the welfare of young children and families is the increasing attention that has been directed to the systematic identification and evaluation of risk conditions that may threaten normal, or even optimal, development (Kopp & Kaler, 1989; Osofsky & Eberhart-Wright, Chapter 2, this volume; Seifer & Sameroff, 1987). For a good many years, infant researchers have been interested in the early detection of developmental delay, particularly with regard to intellectual competence (Wilson, 1985). Infant tests have been used for this purpose, and briefer forms of such tests have been devised for use in wide scale screening for developmental delay (Frankenburg, Emde, & Sullivan, 1985). More recently, some of the newer experimental measures of cognitive functioning in infancy, such as recognition memory or response to novelty, have also been considered as possible screening procedures for identifying infants whose subsequent intellectual development may be compromised (Fagan, Singer, Montie, & Shepherd, 1986; Rose, Feldman, Wallace, & McCarton, 1989). The purpose of such screening, of course, is to allow for consideration of appropriate interventions, which might be applied in the hope of preventing the anticipated delays in development.

A more recent form of screening is aimed at the identification of "risk environments," either in terms of the nature of the overall home environment or in terms of presumably dysfunctional mother-infant relationships. For example, some investigators have been interested in the utilization of an abbreviated questionnaire version of the "HOME" scale (designed to evaluate the home environment) as a screening device (Frankenburg & Coon, 1986). Other investigators in the field have suggested that early-appearing negative maternal attitudes toward their infants, or unfavorable patterns of mother-infant interaction observed early in life, may serve as risk indicators, suggesting the need for early preventive interventions (Lyons-Ruth, Connell, Zoll, & Stahl, 1987; Pianta, Egeland, & Hyatt, 1986).

The social demand for such "environmental" screening methods is likely to continue to increase in the foreseeable future. Consequently, we are likely to see increased research aimed at evaluating the predictive validity of such screening strategies, which is very much needed. Meanwhile, in the absence of obvious and strong evidence of environmental risk to children's health and well-being, the utilization of screening methods of uncertain or very modest predictive validity for identifying families assumed to be at risk and requiring intervention raises difficult ethical as well as scientific questions.

Identification of Cognitive Competencies in Early Infancy

Paralleling the renewed vigor and sophistication with which infants' emotional behavior and development are currently being investigated (as pointed out in Parke's chapter, Chapter 1, this volume), there has been a similar surge of research effort directed at a fuller understanding of the nature and development of various cognitive processes in infancy. Much of this effort has been focused on the identification and measurement of a broader range of cognitive competencies observable as early as the first 6 months of life. There has been considerable emphasis in this research on the predictive value of such assessments and on their potential utilization as early detectors of developmental risk.

One of the areas being most actively investigated is the assessment of visual attentional or information processing behavior, particularly as revealed through habituation-dishabituation paradigms (Sigman, Cohen, Beckwith, & Parmelee, 1986; Tamis-Le Monda & Bornstein, 1989). A number of investigators evaluate infants' attention and information processing through their visual response to novel stimuli in a paired comparison paradigm (Fagan et al., 1986; Rose, Feldman, & Wallace, 1988). With both approaches, encouraging results thus far are reported in terms of positive correlations between these early attentional measures and subsequent IQ scores, suggesting their potential usefulness as predictors of delayed intellectual development.

Several other areas of cognitive functioning are being actively investigated, adding to our understanding of the emergence of significant cognitive competencies very early in infancy. These include systematic studies of early memory (Cutts & Ceci, 1988; Hayne, Rovee-Collier, & Perris, 1987), cross-modal transfer (Rose & Ruff, 1987), and the anticipation of event sequences (Canfield & Haith, 1991; Grace & Suci, 1985).

There is much interest, also, in the processes by which infants "abstract" common properties of visual stimuli, or detect "categories" of such stimuli. Such categorization competencies have been studied in the first 9 to 10 months, primarily through the use of visual habituation and dishabituation methods (Roberts, 1988), or via paired-comparison "novelty preference" procedures (Younger & Gotlieb, 1988). However, as manipulative abilities become more fully developed around the end of the first year, investigators have tended to focus on infant categorization as revealed in object sorting behavior (Goldberg, Starkey, & Fetters, 1982; Sugarman, 1983).

Conclusions

The research trends and anticipated lines of future investigation in infancy research just outlined obviously represent only a part of the picture, although a significant part as viewed from my perspective. There are clearly other emphases and issues of similar importance to current and future research in infant development, and a number of these have been pointed out in the other chapters in this book.

The field of infant research is clearly alive, robust, and growing vigorously. This rapid growth seems at times to be quite fragmented so that there is need both for systematic replication of the many empirical findings reported in our burgeoning journals and for periodic integration of such findings. The importance of moving the field forward in this direction of maturation is highlighted by the fact that most of the significant developmental problems addressed in infant research represent important developmental issues of central concern to the field of human development, or developmental psychology, and not simply to the period of infancy.

References

Allen, D.A., Affleck, G. McGrade, B.J., & McQueeney, M. (1984). Effects of single-parent status on mothers and their high-risk infants. *Infant Behavior and Development, 7*, 347–359.

Anthony, E.J., & Cohler, B.J. (Eds.). (1987). *The invulnerable child*. New York: Guilford.

Beckwith L., & Cohen, S.E. (1984). Home environment and cognitive competence. In A.W. Gottfried (Ed.), *Home environment and early cognitive development* (Chap. 7). New York: Academic Press.

Belsky, J. (1984). The determinants of parenting: A process model. *Child Development, 55*, 83–96.

Bithoney, W.G., & Newberger, E.H. (1987). Child and family attributes of failure-to-thrive. *Journal of Developmental and Behavioral Pediatrics, 8*, 32–36.

Booth, C.L., Lyons, N.B., & Barnard, K.E. (1984). Synchrony in mother-infant interaction: A comparison of measurement methods. *Child Study Journal, 14*, 95–114.

Bradley, R.H., Caldwell, B.M., Rock, S.L., Ramey, C.T., Barnard, K.E., Gray, C., Hammond, M.A., Mitchell, S., Gottfried, A.W., Siegel, L., & Johnson, D.L. (1989). Home environment and cognitive development in the first 3 years of life: A collaborative study involving six sites and three ethnic groups in North America. *Developmental Psychology, 25*, 217–235.

Breitmayer, B., & Ramey, C.T. (1986). Biological nonoptimality and quality of postnatal environment as codeterminants of intellectual development. *Child Development, 57*, 1151–1165.

Bronfenbrenner, U. (1986). Ecology of the family as a context for human development: Research perspectives. *Developmental Psychology, 22*, 723–742.

Canfield, R.L., & Haith, M.M. (1991). Young infants' visual expectations for symmetric and asymmetric stimulus sequences. *Developmental Psychology, 27*, 198–208.

Cocking, R.R. (Ed.). (1986). Issues of early experience in developmental plasticity in cognitive development. *Journal of Applied Developmental Psychology, 7*(special issue), 95–165.

Cohn, J.F., & Tronick, E.Z. (1987). Mother-infant face-to-face interaction: The sequence of dyadic states at 3, 6, and 9 months. *Developmental Psychology, 23*, 68–77.

Cox, M.J., Owen, M.T., Lewis, J.M., & Henderson, V.K. (1989). Marriage, adult adjustment, and early parenting. *Child Development, 60*, 1015–1024.

Crittenden, P.M. (1985). Social networks, quality of child rearing, and child development. *Child Development, 56*, 1299–1313.

Cutts, K.M., & Ceci, S.J. (1988, August). *Memory for Cheerios or Cheerio memory? Long-term retention in young children*. Paper presented at the annual meeting of the American Psychological Association, Atlanta, Georgia.

Drotar, D., & Eckerle, D. (1989). The family environment in nonorganic failure to thrive: A controlled study. *Journal of Pediatric Psychology, 14*, 245–258.

Evans, D.I. (1985). Cerebral function in iron deficiency: A review. *Child care, Health, and Development, 11,* 105–112.

Fagan, J.F., Singer, L.T., Montie, J.E., & Shepherd, P.A. (1986). Selective screening device for the early detection of normal or delayed cognitive development in infants at risk for later mental retardation. *Pediatrics, 78,* 1021–1026.

Fein, G., & Fox, N. (Eds.). (1988). Special issue: Infant day care. *Early Childhood Research Quarterly, 3,* 227–336.

Fox, N.A. (1988) Patterns of brain electrical activity during facial signs of emotion in 10-month-old infants. *Developmental Psychology, 24,* 230–236.

Frankenburg, W.K., & Coon, C.E. (1986). Home Screening Questionnaire: Its validity in assessing home environment. *Journal of Pediatrics, 108,* 624–626.

Frankenburg, W.K., Emde, R.N., & Sullivan, J.W. (1985). *Early identification of children at risk.* New York: Plenum.

Garcia-Coll, C., Vohr, B.R., Hoffman, J., & Oh, W. (1986). Meternal and environmental factors affecting developmental outcome of infants of adolescent mothers. *Journal of Developmental and Behavioral Pediatrics, 7,* 230–236.

Goldberg, S., Starkey, D., & Fetters, L. (1982). Object sorting by preterm and full-term infants. *Infant Behavior and Development, 5*(special ICIS issue), 95.

Gottfried, A.E., & Gottfried, A.W. (Eds.). (1988). *Maternal employment and children's development.* New York: Plenum.

Gottfried, A.W. (1984). Home environment and early cognitive development: Integration, meta-analyses, and conclusions. In A.W. Gottfried (Ed.), *Home environment and early cognitive development: Longitudinal research* (pp. 329–343). New York: Academic Press.

Grace, J., & Suci, G.J. (1985). The role of attentional priority of the agent in the acquisition of word reference. *Journal of Child Language, 12,* 1–12.

Hack, M., & Breslau, N. (1986). Very low birth weight infants: Effects of brain growth during infancy on intelligence quotient at 3 years of age. *Pediatrics, 77,* 196–202.

Hann, D.M. (1989). A systems conceptualization of the quality of mother-infant interaction. *Infant Behavior & Development, 12,* 251–264.

Hayne, H., Rovee-Collier, C., & Perris, E.E. (1987). Categorization and memory retrieval by three-month-olds. *Child Development, 58,* 750–767.

Jacobson, S.W., Fein, G.G., Jacobson, J.L., Schwartz, P.M., & Dowler, J.K. (1985). The effect of intrauterine PCB exposure on visual recognition memory. *Child Development, 56,* 853–860.

Kopp, C.B., & Kaler, S.R. (1989). Risk in infancy: origins and implications. *American Psychologist, 44,* 224–230.

Jones, C.L., & Lopez, R. (1988). *Direct and indirect effects on the infant of maternal drug abuse.* Bethesda, MD: National Institutes of Health.

Lazar, I., & Darlington, R. (1982). Lasting effects of early education: A report from the consortium for longitudinal studies. *Monographs of the Society for Research in Child Development, 47*, (No. 195).

Lyons-Ruth, K., Connell, D.B., Zoll, D., & Stahl, J. (1987). Infants at social risk: Relations among infant maltreatment, maternal behavior, and infant attachment behavior. *Developmental Psychology, 23*, 233–232.

McAnarney, E.R., Lawrence, R.S., Ricciuti, H.N., Polley, J., & Szilagyi, M. (1986). Interactions of adolescent mothers and their 1-year-old children. *Pediatrics, 78*, 585–590.

McCall, R.B. (1983). Environmental effects on intelligence: The forgotten realm of discontinuous nonshared within-family factors.*Child Development, 54*, 408–415.

McCartney, K. (Ed.). (1990). *Child care and maternal employment: A social ecology approach*. San Francisco: Jossey-Bass.

Olson, S.L., Bayles, K., & Bates, J.E. (1986). Mother-child interaction and children's speech progress: A longitudinal study of the first two years. *Merrill-Palmer Quarterly, 32*, 1–20.

Phillips, D. (Ed.). (1987). *Quality in child care: What does research tell us?* Washington, DC: National Association for the Education of Young Children.

Pianta, R.C., Egeland, B., & Hyatt, A. (1986). Maternal relationship history as an indicator of developmental risk. *American Journal of Orthopsychiatry, 56*, 385–398.

Plomin, R. (1989). Environment and genes: Determinants of behavior. *American Psychologist, 44*, 105–111.

Plomin, R., & Daniels, D. (1987). Why are children in the same family so different from one another? *Behavioral and Brain sciences, 10*, 1–60.

Plomin, R., Loehlin, J.C., & De Fries, J.C. (1985). Genetic and environmental components of "environmental" influences. *Developmental Psychology, 21*, 391–402.

Pollack, S., & Vaughn, J. (Eds.). (1987). *Politics of the heart: A lesbian parenting anthology*. Ithaca, NY: Firebrand.

Rauh, V.A., Achenbach, T.M., Nurcombe, B., Howell, C.T., & Teti, D.M. (1988). Minimizing adverse effects of low birthweight: Four-year results of an early intervention program. *Child Development, 59*, 544–553.

Ricciuti, H.N., & Dorman, R. (1983). Interaction of multiple factors contributing to high-risk parenting. In R.A. Hoekelman (Ed.), *Minimizing high-risk parenting* (pp. 187–210). Media, PA: Harwal.

Ricciuti, A.E., & Scarr, S. (1990). Interaction of early biological and family risk factors in predicting cognitive development. *Journal of Applied Developmental Psychology, 11*, 1–12.

Roberts, K. (1988). Retrieval of basic-level category in prelinguistic infants. *Developmental Psychology, 24*, 21–27.

Robertson, S. (1987). Human cyclic motility: Fetal-newborn continuities and newborn state differences. *Developmental Psychobiology, 20*, 425–442.

Rose, S.A., Feldman, J.F., & Wallace, I.F. (1988). Individual differences on infants' information processing: Reliability, stability, and prediction. *Child Development, 59,* 1177–1197.

Rose, S.A., Feldman, J.F., Wallace, I.F., & McCarton, C. (1989). Infant visual attention: Relation to birth status and development outcome during the first 5 years. *Developmental Psychology, 25,* 560–576.

Rose, S.A., & Ruff, H.A. (1987). Cross-modal abilities in human infants. In J.D. Osofsky (Ed.), *Handbook of infant development* (pp. 318–362). New York: Wiley.

Scarr, S., & Ricciuti, A.E. (1991). What effects Do parents have on their children? In L. Okagaki & R.J. Sternberg (Eds.), *Directors of development: Influences on the development of children's thinking.* Hillsdale, NJ: Erlbaum.

Seifer, R., & Sameroff, A.J. (1987). Multiple determinants of risk and invulnerability. In E.J. Anthony & B.J. Cohler (Eds.), *The invulnerable child.* New York: Guilford

Siegel, L.S. (1982). Reproductive, perinatal and environmental variables as predictors of development of preterm (less than 1501 grams) and full terms at 5 years. *Seminar in Perinatology, 6,* 274–279.

Sigman, M., Cohen, S.E., Beckwith, L., & Parmelee, A.H. (1986). Infant attention in relation to intellectual abilities in childhood. *Developmental Psychology, 22,* 788–792.

Sostek, A.M., Smith, Y.F., Katz, K.S., & Grant, E.G. (1987). Developmental outcome of preterm infants with intraventricular hemorrhage at one and two years of age. *Child Development, 58,* 779–786.

Sugarman, S. (1983). *Children's early thought: Developments in classification.* New York: Cambridge University Press.

Tamis-LeMonda, C.S., & Bornstein, M.H. (1989). Habituation and maternal encouragement of attention in infancy as predictors of toddler language, play, and representational competence. *Child Development, 60,* 738–751.

Tinsley, B.J., & Holtgrave, D.R. (1989). Maternal health locus of control beliefs, utilization of childhood preventive health services, and infant health. *Developmental and Behavioral Pediatrics, 10,* 236–241.

Wachs, T.D. (1989). The nature of the physical microenvironment: and expanded classification system. *Merrill-Palmer Quarterly, 35,* 399–420.

Wachs, T.D., & Gruen, G.E. (1982). *Early experience and human development.* New York: Plenum.

Werner, E.E. (1988). Individual differences, universal needs: A 30-year study of resilient high risk infants. *Zero to Three, 8,* 1–5.

Werner, E.E., & Smith, R.S. (1982). *Vulnerable but invincible: A longitudinal study of resilient children and youth.* New York: McGraw-Hill.

Williams, M.L., Lewandowski, L.J., Coplan, J., & D'Eugenio, D.B. (1987). Neurodevelopmental outcome of preschool children born preterm with and without intracranial hemorrhage. *Developmental Medicine and Child Neurology, 29,* 243–249.

Wilson, R.S. (1985). Risk and resilience in early mental development. *Developmental Psychology, 21*, 795–805.

Wolchik, S.A., Braver, S.L., & Sandler, I.N. (1985). Maternal vs. joint custody: children's post separation experiences and adjustment. *Journal of Clinical and Child Psychology, 14*, 5–10.

Woodhead, M. (1988). When psychology informs public policy: The case of early childhood intervention. *American Psychologist, 43*, 443–454.

Youdim, M.B.H., Ben-Shachar, D., & Yehuda, S. (1989). The putative biological mechanisms of the effect of iron deficiency on brain biochemistry and behavior. *American Journal of Clinical Nutrition, 50*, (Suppl.), 607–615.

Younger, B., & Gotlieb, S. (1988). Development of categorization skills: Changes in nature or structure of infant form categories. *Developmental Psychology, 24*, 611–619.

Index